The Carnivore Fix

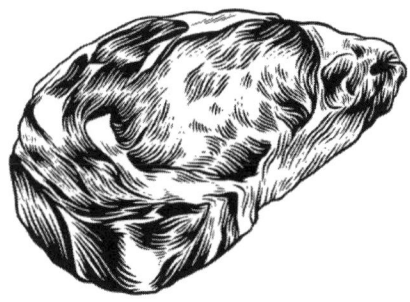

A Comprehensive Guide to a Nose-to-Tail Meat-Based Diet

Dr. Christopher Shaw

Copyright © 2023 - All rights reserved

No part of this book may be reproduced, stored in a retrieval system, or transmitted in any form or by any means, electronic, mechanical, photocopying, recording, or otherwise, without the prior written permission of the copyright owner. The content of this book is protected under international copyright laws and treaties.

Any unauthorized copying, distribution, or dissemination of the material in this book is strictly prohibited and may result in civil and criminal penalties. The author and publisher retain the exclusive rights to the intellectual property contained within this book, including but not limited to text, illustrations, graphics, and layout. Requests for permission to reproduce any part of this book should be addressed to the publisher. Inquiries can be sent to the contact information provided within this book.

Every effort has been made to ensure that the information presented in this book is accurate and reliable. However, the author and publisher make no warranties or representations, express or implied, regarding the completeness, accuracy, or usefulness of the information contained herein. The author and publisher shall not be held responsible or liable for any errors, omissions, or damages arising out of the use of this information.

Trademark names mentioned within this book are the property of their respective owners and are used for identification purposes only. The use of such names does not imply any endorsement, affiliation, or association with the author or publisher.

ISBN: 9798865238928

Disclaimer

The information provided in this book is for educational and informational purposes only. The content is not intended to be a substitute for professional medical advice, diagnosis, or treatment. Always seek the advice of your physician or qualified healthcare provider with any questions you may have regarding a medical condition or before implementing any exercise, dietary, or lifestyle changes. The author and publisher of this book are not responsible for any adverse effects or consequences resulting from the use of the information presented herein. Readers should consult their own healthcare professionals for individualized guidance and recommendations. The author and publisher disclaim any liability for any loss, injury, or damage incurred as a direct or indirect consequence of the use or application of any information provided in this book.

To all those who seek a path less traveled, a return to the wisdom of our ancestors, and a rediscovery of the true nourishment our bodies crave. This book is dedicated to you.

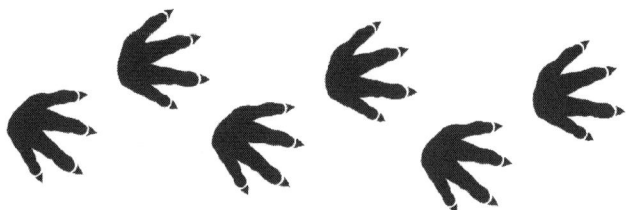

Contents

INTRODUCTION..**15**

CHAPTER 1: CARNIVORE DIET BASICS..........................**19**

Understanding the Carnivore Diet.....................................***19***

   How Often Should You Eat On The Carnivore Diet?.................*23*

   How Much Should You Eat On The Carnivore Diet?...............*24*

   What Negative Symptoms You May Experience When First Starting The Carnivore Diet?..*26*

Carnivore Diet Benefits..***28***

   Weight Loss..*28*

   Decreased Inflammation..*29*

   Increased Testosterone Levels...*30*

   Mental Clarity..*30*

Carnivore Diet Drawbacks...***33***

   Nutrient Deficiencies...*33*

   Lack of Fiber..*34*

   Increased Saturated Fat Intake..*34*

Social Challenges..35

  Long-Term Sustainability...36

Why Plants Are Not Your Friend..38

  Understanding Anti-Nutrients...38

  Types of Anti-Nutrients..41

  Plant-Derived Inflammation and Immunostimulation............50

Nutrients Found Only in Animal Products................................52

  Vitamin B12...52

  Heme Iron...55

  Omega-3 Fatty Acids (EPA and DHA)............................57

  Creatine...59

  Carnitine..61

  Vitamin D3..63

  Choline..66

  Taurine..69

  Vitamin K2..71

  Retinol (Preformed Vitamin A)..74

  Lutein..76

  Astaxanthin...78

  Complete Protein..80

Carnivore Diet Food List...83
Allowable Foods..83
Non-Allowable Foods..85
Carnivore Diet Spices..87
Carnivore Diet Snacks...89
Ask Your Butcher For:..91
Ask Your Fishmonger For:..96
Do You Have to Eat Organ Meats?.....................................100
Is Honey Carnivore?..105
Raw Milk..112

Carnivore Diet Shopping List..117

Carnivore Diet Meal Ideas...119
Breakfasts..119
Snacks...140
Side Dishes..162

7-Day Carnivore Diet Meal Plan....................................175

Eating Out and Traveling on the Carnivore Diet............178
Eating Out on the Carnivore Diet.......................................178
Staying on Track While Traveling......................................179
Examples of What To Order At Restaurants......................180

5 Mistakes to Avoid When First Starting The Carnivore Diet...183

CHAPTER 2: RED MEAT, AN ANCESTRAL NUTRIENT POWERHOUSE..187

Red Meat is Nutritionally Superior to White Meat............190

Are Trans Fats in Red Meat Bad?..191

CLA: How is It Different From Industrial Trans Fats?..........192

Health Benefits of CLA..193

Red Meat: A Great Source of CLA................................196

Common Myths About Red Meat....................................197

Myth 1: Red Meat Causes Heart Disease......................200

Myth 2: Eating Red Meat Causes Cancer......................211

Myth 3: Red Meat Is Inflammatory................................219

Myth 4: Red Meat Causes Kidney Disease in Healthy People..223

Myth 5: Red Meat Causes Gout....................................225

CHAPTER 3: KETO VS. CARNIVORE..231

Exploring the Ketogenic Diet..231

Understanding the Ketogenic Diet................................232

Benefits of the Ketogenic Diet......................................232

Potential Risks and Considerations..............................233

Implementing the Ketogenic Diet..................................240

Similarities and Differences Between the Carnivore and Ketogenic Diets..257

Effects on Metabolic Health and Weight Loss: Which One is Superior?...261

Alternating Between the Ketogenic and Carnivore Diets..266

How To Transition From Keto To Carnivore.......................269

Keto vs. Carnivore: Which One Is Better?..............................271

CHAPTER 4: 40+ CARNIVORE DIET FAQS................274

1. Is the Carnivore Diet Nutritionally Balanced?................275

2. Can the Carnivore Diet Lead to Nutrient Deficiencies?..277

3. What is the Impact of the Carnivore Diet on Gut Health?...280

4. How Does the Carnivore Diet Affect Cholesterol Levels?..282

5. Is the Carnivore Diet Sustainable Long Term?...............284

6. What Are the Potential Risks Associated With the Carnivore Diet?..286

7. Can the Carnivore Diet Be Followed by Athletes or Individuals With High Energy Demands?....................289

8. How Does the Carnivore Diet Impact Blood Sugar Control?...291

9. Are There Any Potential Psychological or Social Implications of Following the Carnivore Diet?............294

10. Is the Carnivore Diet Suitable for Everyone?................296

11. Can the Carnivore Diet Be Sustainable for the Environment?..298

12. Can Children Follow the Carnivore Diet?........................300

13. How to Manage Social Situations and Eating Out While on the Carnivore Diet?..303

14. Can the Carnivore Diet Cause Constipation?..................305

15. Is the Carnivore Diet Suitable for Individuals With Certain Medical Conditions?...308

16. Is the Carnivore Diet Beneficial for Weight Loss?........310

17. Does the Carnivore Diet Have Side Effects?...................312

18. Can the Carnivore Diet Cause Nutrient Excesses?........315

19. Can the Carnivore Diet Cause Digestive Issues?...........317

20. Does the Carnivore Diet Increase the Risk of Cardiovascular Disease?..320

21. Does the Carnivore Diet Increase Testosterone?..........323

22. Can You Build Muscle on the Carnivore Diet?...............325

23. Does the Carnivore Diet Improve Sexual Performance?..327

24. Does the Carnivore Diet Improve Body Composition?..329

25. Does the Carnivore Diet Cause Kidney Problems?.......331

26. How Long Does It Take to Adapt to the Carnivore Diet?..................333

27. What Supplements Should I Take While Following the Carnivore Diet?..................335

28. Does the Carnivore Diet Affect Sleep Quality?..............337

29. Does the Carnivore Diet Make Your Body More Acidic?..................339

30. Does the Carnivore Diet Impair Detoxification?..........341

31. Can the Carnivore Diet Cure Autoimmune Diseases?..342

32. Is the Carnivore Diet Beneficial for Skin Health?........345

33. Is the Carnivore Diet Beneficial for Joint Health?........347

34. Is the Carnivore Diet Beneficial for Hormonal Health?..................349

35. Is the Carnivore Diet Beneficial for Hypothyroidism?..................350

36. Is the Carnivore Diet Good for IBS?...................356

37. Is the Carnivore Diet Good for Psoriasis, Eczema, and Other Autoimmune Skin Conditions?..............358

38. Is the Carnivore Diet Anti-inflammatory?.....................359

39. Why is the Carnivore Diet Considered an Elimination Diet?..................361

40. Is the Carnivore Diet Good for Autism?.........................362

41. Is the Carnivore Diet Beneficial for People With Multiple Food Allergies and Sensitivities?.....................363

CONCLUSION..366

Final Thoughts and Future Directions...................................366

REFERENCES...371

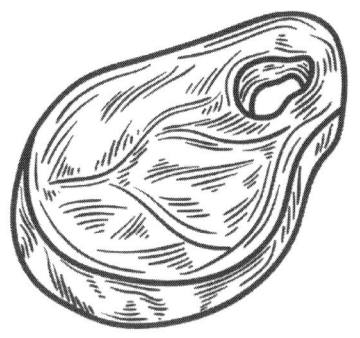

INTRODUCTION

One of the most controversial topics of debate among scientists and the general population alike is what diet is the ideal diet for optimum human health and wellness.

It's estimated that nearly 50% of the American adult population attempts to lose weight at some point every year. Most people recognize that one of the primary ways to lose weight is by changing your diet. Yet, the sheer number of diet plans available makes it extremely challenging to even start, as there is great uncertainty about which one is better, more effective, and sustainable for us.

Every diet seems to have a different objective, with some of them aiming to reduce our appetite, while others suggesting the restriction of certain macronutrients, such as carbohydrates or fats. What's more, many diets seem to offer benefits that go beyond just weight loss.

One such example of a diet with various purported health benefits and applications - from weight loss, improved gut health, optimized body composition, hormonal balance, enhanced mental and cognitive performance, autoimmune healing, etc, that has gained extreme popularity in recent years, is the carnivore diet.

The carnivore diet, as the name implies, is an exclusively animal-based diet that consists entirely of meat and other animal-based products, such as seafood, eggs, and dairy. Animal foods offer a clean, highly bioavailable, and nutritious source of essential dietary components, such as quality proteins, healthy fats, vitamins, minerals, and trace elements, which contribute to human health, longevity, and performance.

This book explores the multifaceted dimensions of the carnivore diet, going beyond just the superficial realms of weight loss and body composition, delving into the unique health advantages of this extreme dietary approach. By picking this book, you willingly embark on a journey to understand the core principles of the carnivore diet: how it works, why, and what can you do to maximize its effectiveness, digging into the scientific research that supports its efficacy, as well as gaining access to countless, amazing, healthy, and delicious recipes.

This book includes a comprehensive overview of the available scientific research on the carnivore diet, allowing you to form informed opinions and make well-founded decisions regarding your diet and health.

Are you ready to embark on such a journey?

If yes, let's start!

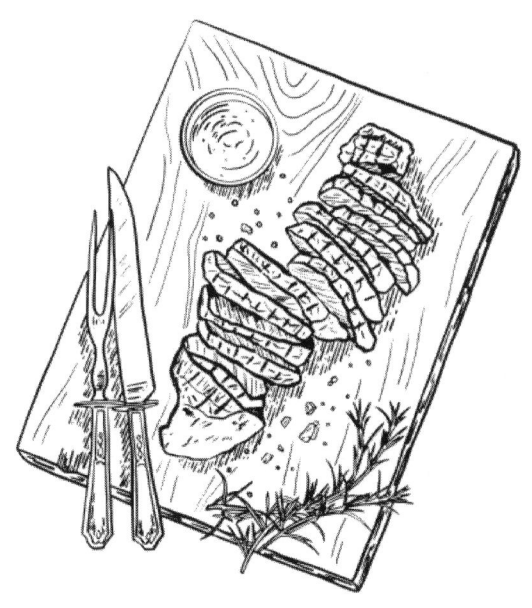

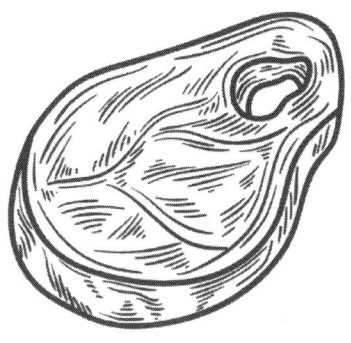

CHAPTER 1: CARNIVORE DIET BASICS

Understanding the Carnivore Diet

The carnivore diet is a meat-based dietary approach that emphasizes the consumption of whole, animal-based foods while excluding all plant foods. This means that your primary sources of energy while on this diet come from protein and fats, while carbohydrates are largely eliminated. By removing plant foods from meals, including fruits, vegetables, nuts, seeds, grains, and legumes, the carnivore diet focuses on animal-based products to fulfil nutrient and energy needs.

The main components of the carnivore diet include red meat, especially fattier cuts, which provide essential micronutrients, such as iron, zinc, creatine, carnitine, selenium, magnesium, and vitamin B12. Organ meats, such as liver, spleen, kidney, and heart, are also favored due to their high nutrient density, offering vital vitamins, minerals, trace elements, and other beneficial compounds like coenzyme Q10 (CoQ10) and choline. Poultry, fish, seafood, and eggs are excellent sources of protein, healthy fats, and essential micronutrients. Animal fats like tallow, lard, and duck fat are also included to provide fuel and nutrients for the body, as well as contribute to satiety. Bone broth, being rich in collagen, minerals, trace elements, and amino acids, as well as bone marrow, a great source of healthy fats and marrow stem cells, are also popular, nutrient-dense additions to the carnivore diet.

Some individuals following the diet may also choose to include full-fat dairy products that are low in lactose, such as hard cheeses, heavy cream, and butter. However, others prefer to exclude dairy altogether due to lactose intolerance, casein sensitivity, or other nutritional concerns. Plant-based beverages, like coffee and tea, are also excluded by strict followers of the carnivore diet, as they are derived from plants. Seasonings like salt and pepper are generally accepted, although some individuals may limit their use to these basics.

Many proponents of the carnivore diet have reported experiencing various positive effects on their health. Accelerated weight loss is often cited as a benefit, which may be attributed to low insulin levels and the diet's emphasis on satiating protein and fat, leading to reduced hunger and overall caloric intake. Improved mental clarity and cognitive function are also commonly reported, potentially due to supplying the brain with missing nutrients, reducing neuroinflammation (inflammation in the nervous system and brain), and eliminating certain plant compounds that could cause inflammation or stimulate the immune system. Better digestion and relief from digestive issues, like bloating, gas, and irritable bowel syndrome (IBS), have been reported by many individuals who have adopted the diet. Additionally, some individuals claim enhanced athletic performance and recovery from exercise while on the carnivore diet.

Overall, the anecdotal evidence from people who have found relief from chronic health issues with this diet is very compelling. For many of them, other dietary approaches had proven ineffective in addressing their chronic health issues, which is quite interesting.

Key Points

• The carnivore diet is a meat-based dietary approach that excludes all plant foods, emphasizing whole, animal-based foods.

• Red meat, including fattier cuts, is a primary component of the carnivore diet, providing essential micronutrients like iron, zinc, creatine, carnitine, selenium, magnesium, and vitamin B12.

• Organ meats such as liver, spleen, kidney, and heart are favored due to their high nutrient density, offering vital vitamins, minerals, trace elements, and beneficial compounds like CoQ10 and choline.

• The carnivore diet is often associated with accelerated weight loss and body recomposition.

• Anecdotal evidence suggests that the carnivore diet has been successful in addressing chronic health issues for many individuals who did not find relief with other dietary approaches.

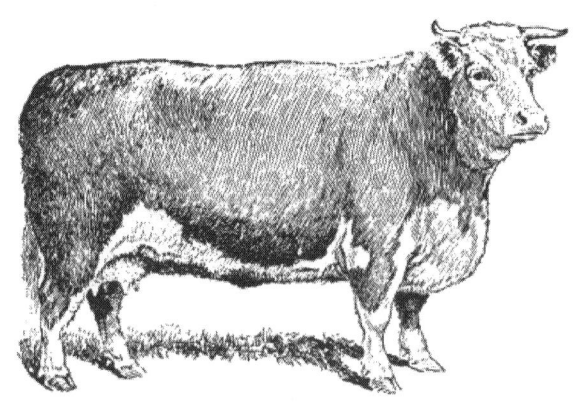

How Often Should You Eat On The Carnivore Diet?

When following the carnivore diet, there are no strict guidelines regarding the frequency of meals. The primary principle is to eat until you feel full and satisfied. This approach allows individuals to tune in to their body's natural hunger and fullness cues, promoting a more intuitive and natural way of eating.

If you prefer to distribute your meals throughout the day, you can choose to have three solid meals or two meals with a snack. This pattern allows for a regular supply of nutrients and energy throughout the day. It can be particularly beneficial for individuals preferring to have consistent meal times or who find it more comfortable to eat at regular intervals.

On the other hand, if you are interested in incorporating intermittent fasting into your carnivore diet routine, you have the flexibility to do so. Intermittent fasting involves periods of fasting followed by eating windows. For example, you may opt for a fasting period of 16 hours, followed by an 8-hour eating window where you consume your meals. This could translate into two meals a day or even one meal a day (OMAD). Intermittent fasting can have various potential benefits, such as improved insulin sensitivity, increased fat burning, and enhanced autophagy (cellular self-cleaning).

For athletes or individuals with increased caloric and nutritional needs, a different approach to meal frequency may be more effective. These individuals may find that spreading their protein intake across two or three meals during the day better supports their athletic performance and muscle recovery. By dividing their meals, they can ensure a consistent and optimal supply of protein and nutrients throughout the day.

Ultimately, the choice of meal frequency on the carnivore diet should be based on personal preference, lifestyle, and individual goals. It is important to listen to your body's signals and adjust your eating pattern accordingly. Experimenting with different meal frequencies and observing how your body responds may help you determine the approach that works best for you.

How Much Should You Eat On The Carnivore Diet?

The carnivore diet emphasizes the principle of eating until you feel full and satisfied, rather than imposing strict portion control. The high satiety value of meat makes it easy to go for extended periods without experiencing hunger pangs. This can be attributed to the slower digestion of meat compared to carbohydrates, which helps regulate cravings and overall food intake throughout the day. Consequently, apart from its potential benefits in reducing inflammation and addressing nutrient deficiencies, the carnivore diet can also be advantageous for individuals aiming to achieve fat loss.

On an average carnivore diet meal plan, approximately two to three pounds of meat are consumed per day. The meat predominantly comes from ruminant, polygastric animals, such as beef, bison, lamb, goat, sheep, or buffalo. During the initial phase of adapting to the carnivore diet, it is not uncommon to consume larger quantities of meat ranging from 4 to 5 pounds per day, as your digestive system and appetite gradually adjust. This adjustment period allows the body to become more accustomed to the absence of other food sources and reduces cravings for non-carnivorous items.

Once you have successfully adapted to carnivore the diet, you may choose to monitor your calorie intake and physical activity levels according to your specific body composition goals. For instance, individuals aiming to build muscle and engaging in regular strength training may find it necessary to consume more fatty meat and dairy products to support their increased caloric and nutritional needs. By tailoring the diet to your specific needs and goals, and tracking relevant factors, you can optimize your results within the framework of the carnivore diet.

It's important to note that while the carnivore diet promotes the consumption of animal-based products, it is still important to prioritize food quality. Opting for grass-fed, organic, and sustainably sourced meats ensures a superior nutrient profile while minimizing potential exposure to harmful substances, such as residues of pesticides, antibiotics, veterinary drugs, and synthetic hormones (i.e. rbGH).

What Negative Symptoms You May Experience When First Starting The Carnivore Diet?

When first starting the carnivore diet, some individuals may experience negative symptoms as their bodies slowly adjust to the new diet. These symptoms are often temporary and may include:

• Brain fog or trouble focusing

• Headaches

• Dehydration

• Mood swings

• Disrupted bowel movements (constipation or diarrhea)

• Nausea

• Indigestion

• Fatigue

• Insomnia

• Dehydration

• Food cravings

It's important to note that individual responses may vary, and these symptoms are not universal. Providing the body with sufficient hydration and electrolytes, such as sodium, potassium, and magnesium, can help mitigate these symptoms during the initial adaptation period.

When transitioning to the carnivore diet, the body undergoes various physiological changes as it adapts to a different macronutrient composition and food sources. The absence of carbohydrates and fiber in the diet may initially impact digestion and bowel movements, leading to constipation or diarrhea in some individuals. This can be attributed to the gut microbiota adjusting to a new dietary environment.

Dehydration is another common symptom during the adaptation phase. The carnivore diet has a diuretic effect, meaning it promotes increased water loss through urine. Therefore, it is crucial to ensure adequate hydration by consuming ample amounts of water throughout the day. Additionally, replenishing electrolytes, such as sodium, magnesium, and potassium, can help maintain proper fluid balance and support optimal bodily functions.

The shift in dietary patterns may also affect mood and energy levels. Some individuals may experience mood swings, fatigue, low energy, or insomnia as their bodies adapt to the absence of carbohydrates or certain food groups, and the adjustment in metabolic processes. These symptoms are normal and transient and typically improve as the body becomes more accustomed to the carnivore diet.

Food cravings, especially for previously consumed carbohydrates, may arise during the initial phase of transitioning to the carnivore diet. This can be attributed to psychological factors, habituation, or the body's adjustment to a completely new dietary pattern. Staying committed to the diet and focusing on the benefits it provides can help overcome these cravings over time.

It's important to approach these potential negative side effects with awareness and patience and allow the body to adapt naturally and gradually. If any concerns persist or worsen, you may consult with a healthcare professional or registered dietitian experienced in low-carb diets, such as keto or carnivore. They will be able to provide personalized guidance and ensure a safe and healthy transition to the carnivore diet.

Carnivore Diet Benefits

The carnivore diet has been associated with various potential benefits related to health, performance, longevity, and overall well-being. Some of these benefits include:

Weight Loss

Similarly to the ketogenic diet, the carnivore diet can lead to significant weight loss due to a shift in the body's primary energy source from carbohydrates to fats. When you consume a strict meat-based diet, your body enters a state of ketosis and becomes fat-adapted. In this state, your metabolism becomes very efficient at utilizing both the fats you consume and your stored body fat as a source of energy. This enables you to burn your own body fat and promotes weight loss.

Moreover, the high-fat and high-protein nature of the carnivore diet promotes long-lasting satiety. Fat and protein are known to be highly filling, which means you can go for extended periods without feeling hungry or the need to consume any food. Additionally, research suggests that becoming fat-adapted can improve the regulation of hunger hormones, helping with appetite control and preventing overeating episodes.

Decreased Inflammation

The carnivore diet has been associated with a potential reduction in inflammation levels, which can have various positive effects on the body. Certain carbohydrate-rich foods, such as those containing refined grains or added sugars, as well as processed foods, have been linked to increased inflammation in the body. Additionally, some plant-based nutrients, while generally beneficial, may trigger inflammatory and/or immune responses in susceptible individuals.

By eliminating these potential sources of food-induced inflammation and focusing on animal-based foods, the carnivore diet can help mitigate inflammation-related symptoms, such as chronic aches and pains. Furthermore, certain protein sources in the carnivore diet, particularly those rich in collagen, contribute to the maintenance and repair of cartilage, the flexible tissue that cushions joints. Improved cartilage health can alleviate joint discomfort and support overall joint function.

Increased Testosterone Levels

The carnivore diet, which emphasizes the consumption of healthy fats and quality proteins, has been associated with potential benefits for testosterone levels. Testosterone is a steroid hormone that plays a crucial role in various aspects of health, including muscle development, strength, energy levels, and overall hormonal balance.

Healthy fats, such as those found in animal foods like meat, fish, eggs, and dairy, are essential for optimal hormone function, including testosterone. Studies have shown that diets rich in healthy fats can support healthy testosterone levels. By following the carnivore diet, which naturally involves an increased intake of healthy fats and protein, individuals may experience improvements in sexual health, muscle mass, strength, and energy levels, commonly associated with high levels of testosterone.

Mental Clarity

Followers of the carnivore diet often report experiencing improved mental clarity, enhanced focus, and increased energy levels. These cognitive benefits can be attributed to several factors associated with the diet.

One significant aspect is the restriction of carbohydrates, which leads to a state of ketosis. When carbohydrates are limited, the body transitions from using glucose (derived from carbohydrates) as its primary fuel source to using ketones, which are produced from the breakdown of fats. This metabolic shift has been shown to have various positive effects on brain function and performance.

Ketones are byproducts of fat metabolism. They have neuroprotective properties and can provide a more stable and efficient energy source for the brain. Unlike carbohydrates, which can result in fluctuations in blood sugar levels and subsequent energy crashes, ketones offer a steady, stable, and consistent energy supply to the brain. This may contribute to increased mental clarity and stamina, focus, and improved cognitive performance.

Additionally, the brain is highly dependent on fats for optimal functioning. Fats are essential for the structure and integrity of cell membranes in the brain, and they play a crucial role in supporting various neurological processes, including neurotransmitter synthesis and signaling. By following a diet that prioritizes healthy fats from whole-food animal sources, such as omega-3 fatty acids found in fatty fish (i.e. salmon, sardines, mackerel, trout, etc), beef brain (great source of DHA), and other animal-based products, individuals on the carnivore diet can provide their brains with the necessary nutrients for optimal cognitive function.

Key Points

• The carnivore diet emphasizes animal-based foods as primary sources of nutrition and energy, focusing on meat (especially red meat), fish, eggs, and dairy.

• The carnivore diet can lead to weight loss by shifting the body's energy source from carbohydrates to fats, promoting fat burning and reducing appetite.

• By eliminating inflammatory foods and focusing on whole, animal-based foods, the carnivore diet can reduce inflammation and alleviate chronic aches and pains. Collagen-rich protein sources, such as bone broth, can also improve connective tissue health.

• The inclusion of healthy fats, quality proteins, and essential micronutrients in the carnivore diet can support optimal testosterone levels, leading to improved muscle mass, strength, libido, and energy.

• The restriction of carbohydrates and the utilization of ketones as a brain fuel source can enhance mental clarity, focus, and cognitive performance. Fats are essential for brain function and neurotransmitter synthesis.

• Ketones derived from fat metabolism have neuroprotective properties and offer a stable and sustained energy supply to the brain, supporting optimal brain function and performance.

• Healthy fats, such as omega-3 fatty acids from animal sources (i.e. fatty fish), are crucial for brain health and cognitive function, as they contribute to cell membrane structure and support neurological processes.

Carnivore Diet Drawbacks

Some potential drawbacks of the carnivore diet may include:

Nutrient Deficiencies

The carnivore diet, characterized by its complete exclusion of plant-based foods, may pose certain challenges in meeting the body's requirements for certain nutrients. Plant-based foods are known to be rich sources of fiber, various vitamins, minerals, trace elements, and antioxidants, which play important roles in maintaining optimal health and well-being.

While animal-based foods provide significant amounts of bioavailable nutrition, such as protein, fats, certain vitamins, minerals, and trace elements, solely relying on them may increase the risk of deficiency in specific dietary constituents found predominantly in plant-based sources. These may include but are not limited to fiber, vitamin C, vitamin E, magnesium, potassium, and various beneficial phytonutrients (i.e. carotenoids, ellagic acid, flavonoids, resveratrol, etc).

Lack of Fiber

Fiber plays a crucial role in digestive health, promoting regular bowel movements, and supporting a healthy gut microbiome. The carnivore diet, which excludes all plant-based sources of fiber, leads to a significant reduction in fiber intake. This can increase the risk of constipation and negatively impact overall gut health. For this reason, individuals following the carnivore diet should prioritize the consumption of organ meats, especially liver (which contains small amounts of animal fiber) and bone broth. These two animal-based foods offer a unique dietary profile that includes essential micronutrients, collagen, and gelatin, which contribute positively to gut health, immune function, and overall metabolism.

Increased Saturated Fat Intake

Animal-based foods, particularly fatty cuts of meat, are known to contain higher levels of saturated fats compared to plant-based foods. Saturated fats have long been associated with an increased risk of cardiovascular disease (CVD) due to their potential to raise blood lipids, specifically low-density lipoprotein (LDL), which is commonly referred to as "bad" cholesterol.

Interestingly, recent scientific studies have sparked debate regarding the relationship between saturated fats and CVD. More and more studies have shown that the link between saturated fat intake and cardiovascular risk is a lot more complex than previously understood. Other factors, such as overall dietary patterns and individual variations in response to saturated fats also play a significant role in CVD risk.

Social Challenges

The carnivore diet can present certain social challenges, as it deviates significantly from conventional dietary patterns. It may be difficult to find suitable meal options when dining out or attending social gatherings, potentially leading to feelings of exclusion or isolation.

One way to navigate these social challenges is through open communication with friends, family, restaurant staff, and healthcare professionals. Explaining the reasons behind your dietary choices and discussing your needs and preferences can help others understand and accommodate your requirements. Sharing your knowledge about the carnivore diet, its potential benefits, and your commitment to your health and/or fitness goals can foster understanding and support from those around you, which is really important and can help you stay on track.

In social situations where you know that food options will be limited, you may take proactive steps. This might involve researching restaurants in advance to identify carnivore-friendly options or communicating your dietary needs to the host when attending social gatherings. Alternatively, you could offer to bring a dish that aligns with your dietary preferences to ensure there is a suitable option available.

Long-Term Sustainability

The long-term sustainability of the carnivore diet is a hot topic of discussion. While anecdotal reports suggest that some individuals can follow the diet long-term, limited official research exists on the potential health risks and benefits of following the carnivore diet over a very extended period of time. Without a diverse range of plant-based foods available, there may be a risk of missing out on certain key phytonutrients and antioxidants, that are associated with various health benefits, such as reducing inflammation, supporting immune function, promoting gut health, and providing protection against chronic diseases. Certain phytonutrients (i.e. carotenoids, ellagic acid, flavonoids, resveratrol, etc) found abundantly in fruits, vegetables, nuts, seeds, and whole grains, have been extensively studied for their positive effects on human health and physiology.

These compounds, including polyphenols, flavonoids, and carotenoids, have demonstrated antioxidant and anti-inflammatory properties, contributing to the prevention of oxidative stress and the promotion of overall health. They have been associated with a reduced risk of conditions, such as heart disease, certain cancers, and neurodegenerative disorders. By excluding plant-based foods, individuals on the carnivore diet may limit their intake of these beneficial phytonutrients, potentially compromising long-term health outcomes.

Key Points

• The carnivore diet may lead to deficiencies in certain nutrients found predominantly in plant-based food sources, such as vitamin C, vitamin E, magnesium, potassium, and various phytonutrients.

• The exclusion of plant-based foods in the carnivore diet results in a significant reduction in fiber intake, which may increase the risk of constipation and negatively impact gut health.

• Animal-based foods, especially fatty cuts of meat, tend to contain higher levels of saturated fats compared to plant-based foods. Excessive intake of saturated fats may have negative effects on cardiovascular health for certain individuals.

• The carnivore diet deviates significantly from conventional dietary patterns, posing challenges when dining out or attending social gatherings. Open communication, proactive planning, and sharing knowledge can help navigate these social challenges and ensure suitable options are always available.

• The long-term sustainability of the carnivore diet is a hot topic of debate. Without a diverse range of plant-based foods, individuals may miss out on important phytonutrients and antioxidants associated with health benefits for human health, including reducing inflammation and supporting immune function. In certain cases, the complete exclusion of plant-based foods may compromise long-term health outcomes.

Why Plants Are Not Your Friend

Plants have long been highly regarded for their nutritional benefits, as they constitute a great source of essential vitamins, minerals, trace elements, fiber, antioxidants, and beneficial phytonutrients.

However, it is important to acknowledge that plants possess certain innate defence mechanisms to protect themselves from pests, diseases, and environmental stressors. These defence mechanisms include the presence of anti-nutrients, compounds that can interfere with the absorption or utilization of nutrients in the human digestive tract.

Understanding Anti-Nutrients

Anti-nutrients are compounds found primarily in plant-based foods, although certain animal foods also contain them (i.e. avidin in egg whites) that can hinder the absorption of nutrients, hence the name "anti-nutrients." In plants, these compounds serve as defence mechanisms against bacterial infections and insects. It's important to understand the different types of anti-nutrients and their potential effects on human health:

- **Glucosinolates and goitrogens:** Found in cruciferous vegetables like broccoli and kale, these compounds can interfere with the absorption of iodine, which may disrupt thyroid function and lead to goiter. People with iodine deficiency or hypothyroidism are particularly vulnerable to these compounds.

- **Lectins:** Lectins are proteins found in legumes and whole grains. They can interfere with nutrient absorption, particularly calcium, iron, phosphorus, and zinc, by binding to these minerals and inhibiting their absorption in the digestive tract.

- **Oxalates:** Oxalates are present in certain foods like green leafy vegetables, tea, beans, nuts, and beets. They can form insoluble calcium oxalate crystals, leading to the formation of kidney stones in genetically-susceptible individuals. Oxalates can also bind to calcium, reducing its bioavailability and absorption.

- **Phytates:** Phytates are naturally occurring compounds found in whole grains, seeds, legumes, and some nuts. They can bind to minerals such as iron, zinc, magnesium, and calcium, reducing their availability for absorption in the digestive system.

- **Saponins:** Saponins are compounds found in legumes and whole grains. They can affect nutrient absorption by disrupting normal digestive processes and potentially causing damage to the lining of the gut.

- **Tannins:** Tannins are present in foods like tea, coffee, and legumes. They can inhibit the absorption of iron by forming complexes with iron and reducing its bioavailability.

The extent of nutrient loss caused by anti-nutrients in our diets is not precisely known and varies among individuals depending on several factors. These factors may include gut health status, genetic makeup, overall diet, cooking and processing methods, and the specific anti-nutrient and food combination.

Many anti-nutrients, such as phytates, lectins, and glucosinolates, can be minimized by soaking, sprouting, or boiling the food before consumption.

It's also important to consider the interaction between anti-nutrients and other nutrients consumed in the same meal in order to minimize their potential negative effects. To reduce the risk, it is advisable to avoid consuming large quantities of foods with anti-nutrients in one sitting and instead opt for a balanced diet throughout the day, incorporating a variety of foods. For example, if having cereal with milk for breakfast, it's recommended to choose a smaller portion of cereal and include fresh berries in the same meal.

Individuals at high risk of diseases related to mineral deficiencies, such as osteoporosis or anemia, may want to monitor their food choices for anti-nutrient content. Modifying the timing of consuming foods with anti-nutrients can also be helpful. For instance, drinking tea between meals instead of with a meal reduces the chances of impaired iron absorption due to the tannins (anti-nutrient) present in the tea. Taking your calcium supplement a few hours after consuming a high-fiber wheat bran cereal containing phytates can also be beneficial instead of taking it at the same time.

While some studies show that vegetarians who consume diets high in anti-nutrient-containing plant foods do not generally experience deficiencies in iron or zinc, other research suggests that their iron stores and blood zinc levels are lower than those of non-vegetarians. The absorption of non-heme iron (the form of iron found in plants) and zinc is influenced by enzyme inhibitors like phytates, which can reduce their absorption by 1% to 23%.

Types of Anti-Nutrients

Lectins

Lectins, also known as hemagglutinins, are a type of anti-nutrient that has gained popularity in recent years. Lectins are present in all plants, but raw legumes (such as beans, lentils, peas, soybeans, and peanuts) and whole grains like wheat contain higher levels of lectins. Some studies suggest that lectins may contribute to gut problems, obesity, chronic inflammation, and autoimmune diseases.

The issue with lectins is that they are proteins that bind to carbohydrates. While they serve as a defence mechanism for plants, their features that protect plants in nature can pose challenges during human digestion. Lectins are resistant to breakdown in the gut and remain stable in acidic environments. When consumed in their active state, lectins can cause adverse effects in humans.

The most widely reported incidents involve severe reactions in people who consume even small amounts of raw or undercooked kidney beans. These beans contain a type of lectin called phytohaemagglutinin, which can cause clumping of red blood cells and lead to symptoms such as nausea, vomiting, stomach upset, and diarrhea. Milder side effects include bloating and gas.

Animal and cell studies have demonstrated that active lectins can interfere with the absorption of minerals, particularly calcium, iron, phosphorus, and zinc. Legumes and cereals, which often contain these minerals, may be affected by the presence of lectins, thereby hindering their absorption and utilization in the body. Lectins can also bind to cells lining the digestive tract, potentially disrupting nutrient breakdown, absorption, and the balance of intestinal flora. Some theories propose that lectins, by binding to cells for extended periods, may trigger autoimmune responses and contribute to inflammatory conditions, such as rheumatoid arthritis and type 1 diabetes.

These theories have sparked a lucrative anti-lectin movement, resulting in best-selling books and enzyme supplements aimed at mitigating lectin activity in the body. However, there is limited research on the amount of active lectins consumed in the diet and their long-term health effects in humans. Studies on anti-nutrients, including lectins, are predominantly conducted in developing countries where malnutrition is prevalent or where food variety is extremely limited, making whole grains and legumes crucial staples in daily meals.

It's important to note that encountering foods with high levels of active lectins is relatively rare. One reason is that lectins are most potent in their raw state, but foods containing lectins are typically not consumed raw. Cooking methods that involve wet heat, such as boiling or stewing, and soaking foods in water for several hours can effectively deactivate most lectins. Since lectins are water-soluble and primarily present on the outer surface of foods, exposure to water helps remove them.

For instance, when preparing dried beans, soaking them for several hours and then boiling them for an extended period softens the beans and disables the lectins. Canned beans are also low in lectins since they are cooked and packaged in liquid. However, raw beans cooked at low heat, such as in a slow cooker, or undercooked beans may still contain lectins.

During digestion, the body can produce enzymes that break down certain lectins. Sprouting grains and beans and mechanically removing the outer hull of beans and wheat grains, which harbor higher lectin levels, are additional processes that can help inactivate lectins.

It's worth noting that different foods contain different types of lectins, and people's reactions to them can vary widely. Individuals with underlying digestive sensitivities, such as irritable bowel syndrome (IBS), may be more prone to experiencing negative symptoms when consuming lectins and other anti-nutrients. If digestive issues arise, it may be reasonable to consume more cooked and processed foods that have lower lectin content. Cooking methods such as boiling, steaming, and baking are effective in reducing lectin levels in various foods. Fermentation, another traditional method of food preparation, can also help to degrade lectins and improve digestibility.

Oxalates

Oxalates are organic compounds classified as antinutrients, commonly found in various plant-based foods, particularly in vegetables like spinach, rhubarb, Swiss chard, and beet greens. These compounds possess strong acidic properties and have the ability to form water-soluble salts by binding to minerals like sodium or potassium and water-insoluble salts by binding to calcium, iron, or zinc.

Historically, dietary oxalate intake has been associated with the pathophysiology of kidney stone disease, a condition characterized by the formation of solid masses called kidney stones within the urinary tract. Human studies have observed a relationship between dietary oxalates and the risk of kidney stone formation. However, it's important to consider that the impact of oxalate content on stone formation differs between soluble and insoluble oxalates. Soluble oxalates, which have a greater bioavailability, are believed to play a more significant role in stone formation compared to insoluble oxalates.

For instance, spinach is known to contain an average of 1145 mg of total oxalate per 100 g of fresh weight, with 803 mg being soluble oxalate. Similarly, almonds have been found to contain 469 mg of total oxalate per 100 g of product, with 153 mg being soluble oxalate. These figures highlight the considerable oxalate content in these foods, especially in terms of their soluble oxalate fractions.

It's worth noting that the impact of dietary oxalate on kidney stone formation may be influenced by other factors as well. Observational studies have shown that individuals with lower dietary calcium intake may be at higher risk of kidney stone formation, whereas those with optimal calcium intake do not exhibit the same increased risk. This has led to the hypothesis that dietary oxalate alone may have minimal impact on kidney stone formation, and ensuring adequate calcium intake should be prioritized instead.

Moreover, research has indicated that the risk of chronic kidney disease progression and end-stage renal disease may be associated with higher levels of urinary oxalate excretion. However, subgroup analyses have suggested that an increased risk of end-stage renal disease was observed only in participants with plasma calcium levels below 9.3 mg/dl, highlighting the complex interplay between oxalates, calcium, and renal health.

While oxalates can potentially contribute to kidney stone formation in susceptible individuals, it is important to consider the overall dietary context, hydration status, and individual factors when evaluating the risk. Maintaining a balanced diet that includes a variety of foods and staying adequately hydrated are crucial strategies for reducing the risk of kidney stone formation.

Phytates

Phytates, also known as phytic acid, are naturally occurring compounds found in high amounts in foods such as nuts, seeds, legumes, and unprocessed whole grains. These compounds have the ability to bind to minerals like iron, zinc, and calcium, forming complexes called phytate-mineral complexes. This binding process can limit the absorption of these minerals in the digestive system, potentially reducing their bioavailability.

The ability of phytates to chelate or bind to minerals has led to concerns about their impact on mineral status and the potential risk of developing mineral deficiencies. In particular, the binding of phytates to iron has received considerable attention. Iron deficiency is a prevalent nutritional problem worldwide, and phytates have been implicated in contributing to iron malabsorption. Similarly, the binding of phytates to zinc and calcium can potentially interfere with the absorption of these essential minerals.

It is important to note that the impact of phytates on mineral absorption is influenced by various factors. For instance, the presence of other dietary components, such as vitamin C (ascorbic acid) or certain organic acids (i.e. citric acid, malic acid, lactic acid), can enhance the absorption of iron in the presence of phytates. Additionally, food processing techniques like soaking, fermenting, or sprouting can help to reduce the phytate content of food and enhance its mineral bioavailability.

Tannins

Tannins are a class of naturally occurring compounds widely distributed in plants. They are particularly abundant in foods such as tea, coffee, certain fruits (i.e. grapes, pomegranates, and berries), and legumes. Tannins are known for their characteristic astringent taste and ability to bind to certain proteins and other organic compounds.

One of the concerns associated with tannins is their potential to interfere with mineral absorption, particularly iron. Tannins can form complexes with iron, reducing its bioavailability and hindering its absorption in the gastrointestinal tract. This has led to concerns about the impact of tannin-rich foods on iron status, especially in populations vulnerable to iron deficiency, such as pregnant women and individuals with low dietary iron intake.

Furthermore, tannins have the capacity to form complexes with other minerals, such as zinc and copper, which may also affect the absorption of these minerals. Prolonged consumption of foods rich in tannins without adequate compensatory measures can increase the risk of mineral deficiencies.

Saponins

Saponins are a diverse group of naturally occurring compounds found in various plants, particularly in legumes, such as beans, lentils, and chickpeas, as well as in certain herbs and vegetables. They derive their name from their ability to produce a soapy foam when mixed with water.

One of the notable characteristics of saponins is their ability to form stable complexes with cholesterol and other lipids. This property has been exploited for their traditional use as natural surfactants and foaming agents in soaps and detergents. However, when consumed orally, saponins can interact with dietary components and physiological processes in the body, leading to potential negative effects on human health.

In terms of their potential impact as anti-nutrients, saponins have been found to interfere with the absorption of certain nutrients, most notably by forming complexes with dietary proteins and inhibiting digestive enzymes (e.g. acting as enzyme-inhibitors). This can affect the bioavailability of certain nutrients, particularly minerals like iron and calcium, leading to decreased absorption and utilization of these essential nutrients.

Protease Inhibitors

Protease inhibitors are naturally occurring compounds that can be found in various foods, with legumes, particularly soybeans, being a notable source. These inhibitors are substances that interfere with the activity of enzymes called proteases, which play a crucial role in breaking down proteins during digestion.

When protease inhibitors are consumed, they can bind to proteases in the digestive system and inhibit their function. This interference can impair the digestion of dietary proteins and potentially reduce the absorption and utilization of essential amino acids, which are the building blocks of protein.

Legumes, such as soybeans, are known to contain relatively high levels of protease inhibitors. However, it is important to note that the effects of these inhibitors can be significantly reduced or minimized through proper cooking and processing methods. Heat treatments, such as boiling or roasting, as well as fermentation and other processing techniques, can deactivate or break down the protease inhibitors, thereby enhancing protein digestibility and availability.

Additionally, the impact of protease inhibitors on protein digestion varies depending on several factors, including the amount consumed, individual differences in enzyme activity, and the overall composition of the person's diet.

Plant-Derived Inflammation and Immunostimulation

Anti-nutrients, found in certain plant-based foods, have garnered attention for their potential role in triggering inflammation and stimulating the immune system in susceptible individuals. These compounds, including lectins, oxalates, phytates (or phytic acid), protease inhibitors, saponins, and tannins, among others, are naturally occurring substances that serve protective functions in plants. While their impact on human health is complex and context-dependent, understanding the mechanisms through which anti-nutrients may influence inflammation and immune function can provide insights into their potential effects.

Interactions with the gut microbiota play a crucial role in modulating immune responses and maintaining gut homeostasis. Anti-nutrients can affect the composition and activity of the gut microbiota, potentially leading to dysbiosis (imbalanced microbial communities) and subsequent immune alterations. For example, lectins have been shown to influence the gut microbiota by binding to specific carbohydrates on the surface of gut bacteria, altering their growth and activity. This disruption in the gut microbial ecosystem can influence the production of metabolites, such as short-chain fatty acids (SCFAs), which have immunomodulatory and anti-inflammatory effects.

Moreover, anti-nutrients can directly interact with immune cells and elicit immune responses. Lectins, a well-studied group of anti-nutrients, have the ability to bind to cell surface receptors on immune cells, including T cells and macrophages. This binding can activate signaling pathways that trigger the release of pro-inflammatory cytokines and chemokines, promoting inflammation. Additionally, lectins may interfere with the functioning of the intestinal barrier, compromising its integrity and potentially allowing the translocation of bacterial components into the bloodstream, further activating immune responses.

The impact of anti-nutrients on inflammation and immune system function is highly individualized, as several factors influence an individual's susceptibility to their effects. Genetic variations in receptor binding sites and immune response genes can determine the degree of immune activation in response to anti-nutrients. Furthermore, gut health plays a crucial role, as a healthy and diverse gut microbiota can provide resilience against potential inflammatory effects of anti-nutrients. A diet rich in fiber and other prebiotics can promote a healthier gut microbiota composition and function, which may help modulate the inflammatory response to anti-nutrients.

The overall dietary pattern also plays a significant role in determining the impact of anti-nutrients on inflammation and immune function. Consuming a varied and balanced diet that includes a wide range of nutrient-dense foods can help mitigate the potential negative effects of anti-nutrients. For instance, cooking, soaking, fermenting, or sprouting certain plant-derived foods can reduce the levels of anti-nutrients and enhance nutrient availability.

Additionally, pairing anti-nutrient-rich foods with other foods that contain specific nutrients can counteract their negative effects. For example, consuming foods rich in calcium, iron, and zinc along with phytic acid-containing foods can help mitigate the mineral-binding properties of phytic acid.

Nutrients Found Only in Animal Products

The debate surrounding the merits of animal-based versus plant-based diets has gained significant attention in recent years. While plant-based diets can provide a wide array of essential dietary components, certain nutrients are exclusively found in animal products. Let's examine some of them:

Vitamin B12

Vitamin B12, scientifically known as cobalamin, is a vital nutrient/water-soluble vitamin that plays a crucial role in various physiological processes in the human body. It is involved in DNA synthesis, the production of red blood cells, and the proper functioning of the nervous system.

When it comes to dietary sources, animal-based foods are the primary providers of vitamin B12. Meat, including beef, poultry, and pork, along with fish, eggs, and dairy products, are particularly rich sources of this important vitamin. These foods contain active forms of vitamin B12 that are readily absorbed and utilized by the body.

Plant-based sources, however, do not naturally contain vitamin B12. This poses a challenge for individuals who follow strict vegan diets, as they exclude animal-based products from their diet altogether. The absence of reliable plant-based sources of B12 increases the risk of vitamin B12 deficiency among vegans.

Insufficient vitamin B12 intake can lead to various health problems. One of the most common consequences is anemia, a condition characterized by a decreased number of red blood cells. Anemia can cause fatigue, weakness, and shortness of breath. In addition to anemia, vitamin B12 deficiency can also result in neurological disorders, including tingling or numbness in the extremities, balance problems, and cognitive impairments.

To ensure adequate vitamin B12 intake, vegans need to pay close attention to their dietary choices and consider appropriate supplementation. Fortified plant-based products, such as plant-based milks, breakfast cereals, and nutritional yeast, are available in the market and can be reliable sources of vitamin B12 for vegans. These fortified products contain synthetic forms of vitamin B12, which are produced through fermentation processes or obtained from bacterial cultures.

Supplementation is another effective way for vegans to meet their vitamin B12 requirements. Vitamin B12 supplements, available in various forms like pills, sublingual tablets, or injections, can provide the necessary doses of this vitamin. It is important for vegans to consult with healthcare professionals or registered dietitians to determine the appropriate dosage and frequency of supplementation based on their individual needs.

Regular monitoring of vitamin B12 levels through blood tests is also recommended to ensure optimal levels and prevent deficiencies. This also allows for adjustments in supplementation dosage or dietary choices if needed.

Key Points

• Vitamin B12 is an essential B complex vitamin crucial for DNA synthesis, red blood cell production, and neurological function.

• Animal-based foods are the primary natural sources of vitamin B12, making it challenging for vegans who exclude these products from their diet to obtain enough amounts.

• Deficiency in vitamin B12 can lead to anemia, neurological disorders, and impaired cognitive function.

• Supplementation and the inclusion of fortified plant-based products are important strategies for vegans to ensure sufficient vitamin B12 intake.

Heme Iron

Iron is an essential mineral that plays a crucial role in various physiological processes in the body, including oxygen transport, energy production, and the synthesis of neurotransmitters. Animal-based products contain heme iron, a form of iron that is more readily absorbed by the body compared to non-heme iron found in plant-based sources.

Heme iron, which is primarily found in animal-based foods such as red meat, poultry, and fish, is highly bioavailable and easily absorbed. It plays a critical role in preventing iron deficiency anemia, a condition characterized by low levels of iron in the body, leading to fatigue, lack of energy, weakness, and impaired cognitive function. Heme iron is particularly important for vulnerable populations, such as pregnant women and children, who have higher iron requirements.

Plant-based sources of iron include legumes, tofu, nuts, seeds, and dark leafy greens. However, the iron found in these sources is non-heme iron, which is not as readily absorbed. Non-heme iron absorption can be influenced by various factors, such as the presence of other dietary components (e.g. vitamin C and certain organic acids, which enhance iron absorption), and the individual's iron status. Although plant-based sources of iron can contribute to overall iron intake, individuals relying solely on plant-based foods may need to pay closer attention to their iron levels and consider additional strategies to ensure adequate iron intake.

For individuals following a plant-based diet, there are several approaches to optimize iron absorption. Pairing plant-based sources of iron with foods rich in vitamin C, such as citrus fruits, berries, and bell peppers, can enhance iron absorption. Cooking plant-based iron sources also improves iron bioavailability. Additionally, avoiding the consumption of substances that are known to inhibit iron absorption, such as tea and coffee (which contain tannins), during meals can help improve iron absorption.

In some cases, individuals relying solely on plant-based foods may find it challenging to meet their iron needs through diet alone. In such situations, iron-fortified products, such as certain cereals, bread, and plant-based milk alternatives, can be a valuable source of supplemental iron. Dietary supplementation may also be considered under the guidance of a healthcare professional or registered dietician, especially for those with known iron deficiency or increased iron requirements (i.e. pregnant women, children).

It is worth noting that iron deficiency can have significant negative health consequences, and individuals following plant-based diets should monitor their iron status through regular blood tests to ensure adequate levels.

Key Points

- Iron is a vital mineral involved in oxygen transport, energy production, and neurotransmitter synthesis.

- Animal-based products provide heme iron, which is more easily absorbed by the body compared to non-heme iron found in plant-based sources.

- While plant-based sources of iron can be included in the diet, individuals relying solely on plant-based foods may need to pay closer attention to their iron intake and consider iron-fortified products or dietary supplementation to ensure adequate iron levels, especially vulnerable populations such as pregnant women and children.

- Regular monitoring of iron status and collaboration with healthcare professionals can help optimize iron intake and prevent iron deficiency anemia in individuals following plant-based diets.

Omega-3 Fatty Acids (EPA and DHA)

Omega-3 fatty acids are essential polyunsaturated fats that are vital for overall health, particularly cardiovascular health, brain function, and inflammation regulation. While plant-based sources such as flaxseeds, chia seeds, and walnuts provide the precursor alpha-linolenic acid (ALA), they do not supply sufficient amounts of the pre-formed, bioavailable, long-chain omega-3 fatty acids eicosapentaenoic acid (EPA) and docosahexaenoic acid (DHA) that are predominantly found in fatty fish and seafood.

EPA and DHA have shown great results in reducing the risk of heart disease, improving cognitive function, and supporting fetal development during pregnancy. They have been extensively studied for their positive effects on cardiovascular health, including reducing triglyceride levels, blood pressure, and inflammation.

While plant-based sources of omega-3s, such as ALA, can be converted into EPA and DHA to some extent, the conversion efficiency is generally limited in the human body. Therefore, individuals following plant-based diets may have lower levels of EPA and DHA compared to those who consume fatty fish and seafood.

To ensure an adequate intake of EPA and DHA, individuals following plant-based diets should consider supplementation with algae-based omega-3 supplements. Algae are the primary source of EPA and DHA in the marine food chain, and algae-based supplements offer a vegan-friendly alternative to fish-derived omega-3 supplements. These supplements are derived from microalgae that naturally produce EPA and DHA.

It is important to note that not all algae-based supplements are the same, and it is advisable to choose high-quality products that have undergone rigorous testing for purity and efficacy. In addition to supplementation, individuals following plant-based diets can improve their omega-3 intake by consuming a well-rounded and varied diet rich in plant-based sources of ALA, such as flaxseeds, chia seeds, hemp seeds, and walnuts. While these sources do not provide significant amounts of EPA and DHA, they still contribute to overall omega-3 intake and offer other health benefits associated with ALA.

Key Points

• Omega-3 fatty acids are essential for cardiovascular health, brain function, and inflammation regulation.

• While plant-based sources provide omega-3s in the form of ALA, they do not supply sufficient amounts of preformed EPA and DHA, which are predominantly found in fatty fish and seafood.

• Individuals following plant-based diets may consider algae-based omega-3 supplements to ensure an adequate intake of EPA and DHA.

• Supplementation, combined with a diet rich in plant-based sources of ALA, can help optimize omega-3 status in individuals who avoid animal-based sources of omega-3s.

Creatine

Creatine is a naturally occurring compound primarily found in animal-based products such as meat (especially red meat) and fish. It plays a crucial role in providing energy to muscles during high-intensity activities. The human body can also synthesize creatine from the amino acids arginine, glycine, and methionine, in the liver, kidneys, and pancreas. However, vegetarians and vegans may have lower levels of creatine in their muscles compared to individuals who consume animal-based products regularly.

Creatine supplementation has gained significant attention in the sports and fitness world due to its well-established ergogenic benefits. Numerous studies have demonstrated that creatine supplementation can increase muscle strength, power, and exercise performance, particularly during short-duration, high-intensity activities, such as weightlifting and sprinting. It works by replenishing the creatine stores in muscles, leading to increased energy production and improved muscle function.

For individuals following a vegetarian or vegan diet, maintaining adequate creatine levels can be achieved through natural synthesis within the body. However, some individuals may choose to supplement with creatine exogenously to optimize their muscle creatine stores and potentially enhance athletic performance. Vegetarian- and vegan-friendly creatine supplements derived from non-animal sources, such as synthetic or plant-based alternatives, are available in the market.

When considering creatine supplementation, it is crucial to choose high-quality products from reputable manufacturers to ensure purity, efficacy, and safety. Additionally, proper dosing guidelines and recommendations should be followed to avoid potential side effects or adverse reactions. Adequate hydration and regular monitoring of kidney function are also important factors to consider while using creatine supplements.

Key Points

• Creatine is a naturally occurring compound found primarily in meat (especially red meat) and fish. It plays a vital role in providing energy to muscles during high-intensity physical activities.

• While vegetarians and vegans have lower creatine levels than meat eaters, they may be able to maintain adequate levels through natural synthesis within their body and by considering creatine supplements derived from non-animal sources.

• Creatine supplementation has been shown to enhance muscle strength, power, and performance, particularly during short-duration, high-intensity activities.

• Before starting any supplementation regimen, including creatine, individual needs and goals should be taken into account, and consultations with healthcare professionals or registered dietitians may be necessary.

Carnitine

Carnitine is an amino acid-like compound that plays a crucial role in the transport of fatty acids into the mitochondria, the energy-producing organelles of cells. It facilitates the conversion of fatty acids into usable energy through a process known as beta-oxidation. Carnitine is predominantly found in animal-based foods, with meat and dairy being the richest dietary sources.

The human body can synthesize small amounts of carnitine from the amino acids lysine and methionine. However, endogenous production may not be sufficient to meet the body's needs, particularly in the presence of certain medical conditions (i.e. primary or secondary carnitine deficiency) or dietary restrictions. Strict vegetarians and vegans who exclude animal-based products from their diet may have lower levels of carnitine compared to individuals who consume animal products regularly.

Carnitine deficiency can have negative effects on fat metabolism and energy production. It may lead to reduced ability to utilize fatty acids as an energy source, resulting in muscle weakness, fatigue, and impaired exercise performance. In some cases, carnitine supplementation may be warranted to ensure adequate carnitine levels and support optimal energy metabolism.

For individuals following plant-based diets, maintaining sufficient carnitine levels can often be achieved through efficient endogenous synthesis. The body has the ability to upregulate carnitine synthesis to compensate for lower dietary intake. However, certain factors such as age, health status, and physical activity levels can influence the body's ability to synthesize carnitine.

In cases where individuals may require additional carnitine supplementation, vegetarian and vegan-friendly carnitine supplements derived from non-animal sources are available. These supplements typically contain L-carnitine or its derivatives, which can be effectively absorbed and utilized by the body.

Key Points

• Carnitine is an amino acid-like compound primarily found in meat and animal products. It plays a vital role in the transport of fatty acids into the mitochondria for energy production.

• While the body can synthesize carnitine to some extent, individuals following plant-based diets may need to pay closer attention to their carnitine status.

• Efficient endogenous synthesis and a well-planned plant-based diet can oftentimes maintain sufficient carnitine levels in the body.

• In certain cases, within the context of a plant-based diet, carnitine supplementation derived from non-animal sources may be considered under the guidance of a healthcare professional or registered dietitian.

Vitamin D3

Vitamin D is a crucial fat-soluble vitamin/prohormone with a wide range of physiological functions. It plays a vital role in bone health, immune function, and the regulation of various cellular processes in the body.

Animal-based sources are known to be rich in vitamin D, particularly vitamin D3 (cholecalciferol), which is the active form of the vitamin. Fatty fish, such as salmon, mackerel, and sardines, are excellent sources of vitamin D3. Fish liver oils, such as cod liver oil, are also highly concentrated sources. Additionally, egg yolks contain small amounts of vitamin D3.

Plant-based sources mainly provide vitamin D2 (ergocalciferol). Certain types of mushrooms, such as shiitake and maitake mushrooms, can synthesize vitamin D2 when exposed to ultraviolet (UV) light. Fortified plant-based foods, including some plant-based milks, breakfast cereals, and juices, may also contain added vitamin D2.

Both vitamin D2 (ergocalciferol) and vitamin D3 (cholecalciferol) can be converted to the active form of vitamin D in the body (calcitriol). However, some research suggests that vitamin D3 may be more effective in raising blood levels of vitamin D than vitamin D2. This is due to differences in their metabolism and binding affinity to vitamin D receptors.

Individuals following plant-based diets, especially strict vegan diets, should be mindful of their vitamin D status and take steps to ensure adequate levels. Sunlight exposure is an excellent natural source of vitamin D, as the skin can synthesize it when exposed to UVB rays. However, factors such as geographical location, season, skin pigmentation, and the use of sunscreen can affect the body's ability to produce vitamin D from sunlight.

Fortified foods can be an important source of vitamin D for individuals following plant-based diets. Consuming plant-based milks, breakfast cereals, and other fortified products that contain vitamin D2 or vitamin D3 can help meet daily requirements. It is important to check product labels for the specific type and amount of vitamin D provided.

If obtaining sufficient vitamin D through sunlight and fortified foods is a challenge, individuals may consider vitamin D3 supplements. These supplements, oftentimes derived from animal-based sources, like lanolin (natural wax-like substance derived from sheep wool), can help maintain optimal vitamin D levels. However, it is recommended to consult with healthcare professionals or registered dietitians to determine the appropriate dosage and duration of vitamin D3 supplementation.

Regular monitoring of vitamin D levels through blood tests is also advisable to ensure adequate intake and prevent deficiencies.

Key Points

- Vitamin D3 (cholecalciferol) is the active form of vitamin D found in animal-based sources like fatty fish, fish liver oils, and egg yolks.

- Plant-based sources primarily provide vitamin D2 (ergocalciferol) found in certain mushrooms and fortified plant-based foods.

- Both vitamin D2 and D3 can be converted to the active form of vitamin D in the body, called calcitriol.

- Research suggests that vitamin D3 may be more effective than vitamin D2 in raising blood levels of vitamin D due to differences in metabolism and binding affinity to receptors.

• Individuals following plant-based diets should ensure adequate vitamin D levels through sunlight exposure, fortified foods, or consider vitamin D3 supplementation under professional guidance. Regular monitoring of vitamin D levels is advisable.

Choline

Choline is a water-soluble vitamin-like compound with critical roles in various aspects of human health and physiology. While not technically classified as a vitamin, it is often grouped with the B-vitamins due to its similar functions and importance in the body. Choline is vital for various physiological processes, including cell structure, nerve function, metabolism, and the synthesis of neurotransmitters. It is involved in the formation of phospholipids, which are essential components of cell membranes, and acts as a precursor for the neurotransmitter acetylcholine. Choline is particularly important during pregnancy and early childhood due to its impact on brain development and cognitive function.

While some plant-based sources contain choline, such as soybeans and cruciferous vegetables (i.e. broccoli, Brussels sprouts, etc), they generally provide lower amounts compared to animal-based sources. Animal-based foods, such as eggs, liver, and meat, are considered particularly rich sources of choline.

Eggs, especially the yolk, are one of the best sources of dietary choline. In fact, one large egg can provide around 147 milligrams of choline, which is more than a quarter of the recommended daily intake (RDI) for adults. Liver, both from poultry and beef, is another animal-based food known for its high choline content. Meat, including beef, pork, and poultry, also contains notable amounts of choline.

Adequate choline intake is essential for various physiological functions. During pregnancy, choline plays a crucial role in fetal brain development, including neural tube formation and memory enhancement. Studies have shown that higher maternal choline intake during pregnancy is associated with improved cognitive function and decreased risk of neural tube defects in infants.

In early childhood, choline continues to support brain development and cognitive function. It contributes to the production of acetylcholine, a neurotransmitter that plays a role in memory, learning, and muscle control. Choline also influences liver function by aiding in the metabolism of fats and cholesterol.

While plant-based sources of choline exist, individuals following strict vegan or plant-based diets should pay close attention to their choline intake. They may need to incorporate a variety of choline-rich plant-based foods into their diet or consider choline supplements to meet their needs, especially during critical periods such as pregnancy and early childhood.

It is worth noting that the choline content of foods can vary depending on factors such as farming practices, feed composition, and cooking methods. Therefore, it is essential to choose high-quality sources of animal-based products and prepare them in ways that retain their nutrient content. This ensures that you obtain optimal levels of choline. Additionally, incorporating a wider variety of animal-based products in your diet can provide a broader spectrum of nutrients, including choline, helping you achieve nutritional balance.

Key Points

• Choline is a water-soluble vitamin-like compound important for cell structure, nerve function, metabolism, and neurotransmitter synthesis.

• Animal-based sources such as eggs, liver, and meat are rich in choline compared to plant-based sources.

• Adequate choline intake is crucial during pregnancy and early childhood for brain development and cognitive function.

• Individuals following strict vegan or plant-based diets should be mindful of their choline intake and may need to incorporate choline-rich plant-based foods or consider supplements.

• The choline content of foods can vary, so choosing high-quality animal-based products and preparing them properly helps ensure optimal choline intake.

Taurine

Taurine is an amino acid-like compound that is involved in various physiological processes in the body. Although it is not technically classified as an amino acid, it shares some similarities with amino acids in its structure and functions.

Taurine plays a role in bile acid conjugation, which is important for the digestion and absorption of dietary fats. It is also known for its antioxidative properties, helping to protect cells from oxidative stress and damage.

Taurine is also involved in osmoregulation, as it helps regulate the balance of water and electrolytes in cells. It acts as an osmolyte, helping to maintain cell volume and fluid balance.

Additionally, taurine partakes in the modulation of cellular calcium levels, which is important for proper muscle function, neurotransmission, and other cellular processes.

Although taurine can be synthesized by the body from the amino acids cysteine and methionine, animal-based foods are the primary dietary sources of this compound. Meat, particularly beef and poultry, along with seafood and dairy products, are known to contain significant amounts of taurine. These foods provide an easily absorbable form of taurine, ensuring sufficient intake for individuals who include them in their diet.

For vegetarians and vegans who exclude animal-based products from their diet, maintaining adequate levels of taurine can be a challenge. However, studies have shown that the body can synthesize taurine endogenously from the sulfur-containing amino acids methionine and cysteine. As long as vegetarians and vegans consume a well-balanced diet with sufficient protein intake, their bodies may be able to synthesize the required amounts of taurine.

It's worth noting that certain factors may affect endogenous taurine production. For instance, individuals with specific health conditions (i.e., liver disease) or those on restricted diets (i.e., vegan or vegetarian diets) may have altered taurine synthesis capabilities. In such cases, it may be advisable to consult with a healthcare professional or registered dietitian to assess the need for taurine supplementation.

While taurine is not considered an essential nutrient since the body can synthesize it on its own, some research suggests potential benefits of taurine supplementation in certain circumstances. Particularly, taurine supplementation has been studied for its potential role in supporting cardiovascular health, regulating blood sugar levels, and improving exercise performance. However, more research is needed to fully understand the extent of these effects and the specific populations that may benefit from taurine supplementation.

Key Points

• Taurine is an amino acid-like compound involved in various physiological processes in the body, including bile acid conjugation, antioxidative protection, osmoregulation, and cellular calcium modulation.

• Animal-based foods, such as meat, seafood, and dairy products, are the primary dietary sources of taurine.

• Vegetarians and vegans can synthesize taurine endogenously from methionine and cysteine if they maintain a well-balanced diet with sufficient protein intake.

• Certain health conditions, like liver disease, or restricted diets, such as vegan or vegetarian diets, may impact the body's taurine synthesis capabilities.

• Taurine supplementation has potential benefits for cardiovascular health, blood sugar regulation, and exercise performance, but further research is needed to understand the extent and specific populations that may benefit.

Vitamin K2

Vitamin K is a vital fat-soluble vitamin that plays a crucial role in blood clotting and bone health. It exists in two main forms: vitamin K1 (phylloquinone) and vitamin K2 (menaquinone).

Animal-based foods, especially certain types of fermented and aged cheeses, are known to be rich sources of vitamin K2. They contain specific strains of bacteria that produce vitamin K2 during the fermentation process. Vitamin K2, specifically the longer-chain menaquinones (MKs), has been shown to have a more significant impact on bone health compared to vitamin K1.

On the other hand, most plant-based sources provide vitamin K1. Leafy green vegetables, such as spinach, kale, and broccoli, are particularly abundant in vitamin K1. While vitamin K1 is not as readily utilized by the body for bone health as vitamin K2, it is still important for blood clotting and overall vitamin K status.

Both vitamin K1 and vitamin K2 contribute to maintaining adequate vitamin K levels in the body. Vitamin K is involved in the activation of proteins involved in blood clotting, which is essential for the proper functioning of the coagulation cascade. Additionally, vitamin K is also involved in regulating calcium metabolism and bone health by activating proteins that help transport and incorporate calcium into bone tissues.

While vitamin K2 has demonstrated a more significant impact on bone health, individuals following plant-based diets can still obtain sufficient vitamin K1 by consuming a variety of leafy green vegetables and other plant-based sources. It is important to note that the conversion of vitamin K1 (phylloquinone) to vitamin K2 (menaquinone) in the body is limited, and direct dietary sources of vitamin K2 are primarily derived from animal-based foods, except for natto - a traditional Japanese food made from fermented soybeans.

For individuals who exclude animal-based products from their diet, it may be beneficial to consider other strategies to support bone health. These strategies may include optimizing vitamin D levels, as vitamin D works synergistically with vitamin K2 in maintaining proper calcium balance in the body. Additionally, fermented plant-based foods such as sauerkraut and certain types of plant-based cheeses may provide small amounts of vitamin K2 due to the presence of specific bacteria that produce it.

Key Points

• Vitamin K is involved in blood clotting, calcium metabolism, and bone health by activating proteins that transport and incorporate calcium into bone tissues.

• Vitamin K2, particularly the longer-chain menaquinones (MKs), has a more significant impact on bone health compared to vitamin K1.

• Animal-based foods, including certain fermented and aged cheeses, are rich sources of vitamin K2.

• Plant-based sources, such as leafy green vegetables, provide vitamin K1, which is important for blood clotting and overall vitamin K status.

- The conversion of vitamin K1 to vitamin K2 in the body is limited, and direct dietary sources of vitamin K2 are primarily derived from animal-based foods, except for natto - a fermented soybean food of Japanese origin.

Retinol (Preformed Vitamin A)

Retinol, the preformed and active form of vitamin A, is a vital fat-soluble vitamin that plays a crucial role in various physiological processes in the body, including vision, immune function, and cellular differentiation. While animal-based sources are rich in retinol, plant-based foods provide provitamin A carotenoids, such as beta-carotene, which can be converted by the body into retinol to some extent.

Animal-based sources of retinol include liver, fish, eggs, dairy products, and animal-based oils (i.e. fish oil, cod liver oil, etc). These foods contain readily available retinol, which can be directly utilized by the body. Retinol is important for vision as it is a key component of the visual pigment in the retina, known as rhodopsin. It is also involved in maintaining healthy immune function and promoting proper cellular differentiation, which is essential for growth and development.

Plant-based sources, on the other hand, offer provitamin A carotenoids, such as beta-carotene, alpha-carotene, beta-cryptoxanthin, and lycopene. These carotenoids are pigments found in certain fruits and vegetables, particularly in orange, yellow, red, and dark green varieties. Beta-carotene is the most well-known provitamin A carotenoid. The body can convert provitamin A carotenoids into retinol, but the efficiency of this conversion can vary among individuals. Factors such as genetics, dietary composition, and overall health can influence the conversion process.

Individuals following plant-based diets should ensure an adequate intake of provitamin A carotenoids to meet their vitamin A needs. Good sources of beta-carotene include carrots, sweet potatoes, dark leafy greens like spinach and kale, and orange-colored fruits like mangoes and apricots. These foods provide the precursors necessary for the body to synthesize retinol.

It is worth noting that the conversion efficiency of provitamin A carotenoids to retinol is generally lower than the absorption efficiency of preformed retinol from animal-based sources. Therefore, individuals following plant-based diets, especially those with limited intake of animal-based foods, should pay close attention to their vitamin A status and consider factors that may affect conversion efficiency.

To optimize the conversion of provitamin A carotenoids into retinol, it is advisable to consume foods rich in healthy fats along with provitamin A sources. Fats have been shown to enhance the absorption and utilization of carotenoids. Including sources of healthy fats like avocados, nuts, seeds, and oils can support this conversion process.

Key Points

• Retinol is the active form of vitamin A and is found in animal-based sources such as liver, fish, eggs, dairy products, and animal-based oils.

• Retinol plays a crucial role in vision, immune function, and cellular differentiation.

• Plant-based foods provide provitamin A carotenoids like beta-carotene, which can be converted into retinol to some extent.

• Good sources of provitamin A carotenoids include carrots, sweet potatoes, dark leafy greens, and orange-colored fruits.

• The conversion efficiency of provitamin A carotenoids to retinol is generally lower than the absorption efficiency of preformed retinol from animal-based sources. However, including healthy fats in the diet can support the conversion process.

Lutein

Lutein is a carotenoid pigment that plays a crucial role in promoting eye health. It acts as a powerful antioxidant, protecting the retina and lens from oxidative damage and maintaining optimal visual function. Lutein is associated with reducing the risk of age-related macular degeneration (AMD) and cataracts, common eye conditions that can impair vision.

Animal-based sources, such as egg yolks and certain animal fats, are rich in lutein. These sources provide highly bioavailable lutein, meaning it is easily absorbed and utilized by the body. Egg yolks, in particular, are known for their concentrated lutein content.

Plant-based sources of lutein include dark leafy greens like spinach, kale, and collard greens. While these vegetables contain lutein, its bioavailability from plant-based sources is lower compared to animal sources. Factors like food preparation, cooking methods, and the presence of dietary fats can influence lutein absorption. Pairing lutein-rich vegetables with sources of dietary fat, such as olive oil or avocado, can enhance lutein absorption.

To ensure sufficient lutein intake for optimal eye health, it is recommended to consume a combination of animal-based and plant-based sources. Including foods like egg yolks, animal fats, and dark leafy greens in the diet provides a diverse range of lutein sources. Dietary supplements containing lutein derived from various sources, including marigold flowers, are also available for those who may have difficulty obtaining enough lutein through diet alone.

Key Points

• Lutein is a carotenoid and antioxidant that plays a critical role in promoting eye health, particularly in protecting against age-related macular degeneration (AMD) and cataracts.

• Animal-based sources, such as egg yolks and certain animal fats, are rich in lutein and highly bioavailable. Plant-based sources, such as dark leafy greens, also contain lutein, although their bioavailability is lower.

• A combination of animal-based and plant-based sources can help ensure adequate lutein intake for optimal eye health.

• As part of a comprehensive eye care approach, incorporating lutein-rich foods and, if necessary, considering lutein supplements can be beneficial.

Astaxanthin

Astaxanthin is a vibrant red pigment and powerful antioxidant that offers a wide range of health benefits. It is a carotenoid compound that is naturally produced by certain types of microalgae, and it accumulates in the tissues of marine animals that consume these algae. Animal-based sources, particularly those derived from marine sources, are considered the primary dietary sources of astaxanthin.

The rich red hue of marine animals like salmon, trout, and shrimp is attributed to the presence of astaxanthin in their tissues. These animals obtain astaxanthin through their diet, as they consume the microalgae that produce this pigment. By consuming marine-derived animal-based products, individuals can obtain a more concentrated source of astaxanthin.

Astaxanthin is renowned for its potent antioxidant benefits, which help to combat oxidative stress and reduce inflammation in the body. It has been studied for its potential benefits in various areas, including cardiovascular health, eye health, immune function, and cognitive performance. Astaxanthin is also known for its neuroprotective properties, which may contribute to its potential role in supporting brain health.

While plant-based sources like red-pinkish fruits (i.e. red berries, red-pink grapefruit) do contain small amounts of astaxanthin, the levels are significantly lower compared to animal-based sources. Plant-derived astaxanthin is generally considered to be less bioavailable and less concentrated. Therefore, to obtain higher levels of astaxanthin, incorporating marine-derived animal-based products into the diet is recommended.

It's important to note that astaxanthin is not considered an essential nutrient, as the body is not able to synthesize it. However, its potential health benefits and powerful antioxidant properties make it an intriguing compound worthy of attention. Astaxanthin supplements derived from microalgae are available for those who may want to ensure sufficient intake, especially if they do not consume animal-based products.

Key Points

• Astaxanthin is a red pigment and powerful antioxidant.

• High levels of bioavailable astaxanthin are primarily found in marine-derived animal-based sources, such as salmon, trout, and shrimp.

• Plant-based sources do contain astaxanthin in smaller amounts, but the levels are significantly lower and less bioavailable.

• Astaxanthin offers various health benefits, including anti-inflammatory and neuroprotective properties.

• Individuals who do not consume animal-based products may consider astaxanthin supplements derived from microalgae as an alternative.

Complete Protein

Protein is an essential macronutrient that plays a fundamental role in numerous physiological processes in the body. It is involved in growth and development, tissue repair, enzyme production, hormone synthesis, and the maintenance of a healthy immune system. While protein can be obtained from both animal-based and plant-based sources, there are some notable differences to consider.

Animal-based products are considered complete proteins because they contain all the essential amino acids required by the human body in adequate proportions.

Essential amino acids are those that the body cannot produce on its own and must be obtained through the diet. Examples of animal-based protein sources include meat, poultry, fish, eggs, and dairy products. These sources offer a wide range of essential amino acids and are highly bioavailable, meaning they are readily absorbed and utilized by the body.

In contrast, plant-based protein sources often lack one or more essential amino acids, and thus are considered incomplete proteins. That is an important difference, however, it does not necessarily mean that plant-based protein sources are insufficient or inferior. With proper planning and dietary variety, individuals following vegan or vegetarian diets can still obtain all the essential amino acids they need. By combining different plant protein sources throughout the day, such as legumes, whole grains, nuts, and seeds, it is possible to achieve a complete amino acid profile.

In the past, it was a common belief that specific combinations of plant proteins had to be consumed at the same meal to ensure a complete amino acid profile. This concept, known as protein combining or complementary protein, suggested that certain plant proteins needed to be consumed together to compensate for the lacking amino acids in one source. However, recent research has shown that the body is capable of utilizing amino acids from various meals throughout the day, and the importance of precise protein combining is less important than previously thought. A varied and balanced plant-based diet that includes a wide range of protein sources can still provide sufficient protein intake and meet the body's amino acid requirements.

It is worth noting that individual protein needs can vary based on factors such as age, sex, body weight, physical activity level, and overall health status. Consulting with a healthcare professional or registered dietitian can provide personalized guidance on protein intake and dietary considerations.

Key Points

• Protein is an essential macronutrient involved in countless physiological functions in the body.

• Animal-based proteins are considered complete proteins, providing all the essential amino acids in adequate proportions.

• Plant-based protein sources lack certain essential amino acids (i.e. lysine, methionine, tryptophan, threonine, isoleucine, valine), but by incorporating a variety of plant proteins throughout the day (not necessarily in the same meal), individuals following vegan or vegetarian diets can still achieve a complete amino acid profile.

• The concept of precise protein combining in every meal is now considered outdated, and a varied and balanced plant-based diet may still provide sufficient protein intake.

Carnivore Diet Food List

The carnivore diet allows and prohibits the following foods:

Allowable Foods

On the carnivore diet, the following foods are allowed:

- **Meat:** Focus on fatty cuts of grass-fed red meat, such as ribeye steak, prime rib, brisket, T-bone, etc. The higher fat content in these cuts provides more energy/calories and essential micronutrients, including fat-soluble vitamins A, D, E, and K. These vitamins are important for various physiological processes in the body and promote overall health.

- **Fish:** Opt for wild-caught, fatty fish, like salmon, sardines, trout, and mackerel. These types of fish are rich in omega-3 fatty acids (EPA and DHA), which have been associated with numerous health benefits, including cardiovascular health, brain health, joint health, and inflammation regulation.

- **Eggs:** Considered "nature's multivitamin," eggs are a balanced source of protein, fats, and essential micronutrients, including vitamins, minerals, trace elements, and antioxidants. They are highly nutritious and provide a variety of nutrients needed for optimal health and wellness.

- **Bone Broth:** Bone broth provides highly bioavailable protein and collagen. It is rich in amino acids and minerals, which support gut health, skin health, immune function, and the health of connective tissues and joints.

- **Dairy:** Organic full-fat milk (especially raw milk), grass-fed butter, cream, yogurt, kefir, and cheese are allowed on the carnivore diet. However, some people choose to limit or avoid dairy due to potential intolerances or allergies. Dairy products can be a good source of quality protein, healthy fats, and certain vitamins and minerals, like sodium, calcium, potassium, magnesium, and phosphorus.

- **Animal-Based Fats and Oils:** Use animal-based fats, like lard, tallow, and duck fat, for cooking instead of vegetable oils. These fats are more stable at high temperatures and provide excellent sources of micronutrients, especially fat-soluble vitamins A, D, E, and K. You may also supplement with animal-based oils, like fish oil or cod liver oil, to supply your body with large amounts of beneficial omega-3 fatty acids.

- **Spices and Seasonings:** Salt, pepper, herbs, and spices without sugar or carbohydrates can be used to enhance the flavor of dishes and meals. These spices and seasonings add variety and taste to food while keeping the diet animal-based.

Non-Allowable Foods

On the carnivore diet, the following foods are not allowed:

• **Fruits:** All fruits, including apples, bananas, oranges, berries, and tomatoes, are excluded. This is because fruits contain natural sugars (especially fructose) and carbohydrates that are not part of the carnivore diet's focus on low-carb eating. Additionally, some fruits contain harsh fibers and anti-nutrients that can irritate the gut, contribute to inflammation, and stimulate the immune system.

• **Vegetables:** All vegetables, including broths and condiments made from vegetables, are not allowed. Vegetables are typically high in fiber, carbohydrates, and various anti-nutrients, which should be avoided while on the carnivore diet.

• **Added Sugars:** Any form of added sugars is not allowed on the carnivore diet. Simple sugars stimulate insulin and impair metabolic health. Limiting insulin spikes contributes to restoring insulin sensitivity and improves metabolic health. One of the primary objectives of the carnivore diet is to heal the metabolism.

• **Additives:** Processed foods (even processed meat products, like deli meats) with additives like soy protein isolate, nitrates, nitrites, artificial sweeteners, and MSG (monosodium glutamate) are not allowed on the carnivore diet. These compounds are inflammatory, overexcite the nervous system, disrupt the natural balance of the gut microbiome, impair cellular function and communication, and can stimulate the immune system.

• **Low-Quality Meats:** Conventional, grain-fed meats are not excluded from the carnivore diet (many people can't afford or don't have access to organic); however, they are not preferred over their organic, grass-fed counterparts. Organic, grass-fed, pasture-raised meats are more nutrient-dense and contain fewer toxins, including residues of antibiotics, veterinary drugs, and hormones, that typically accumulate in the fatty tissues of conventionally-raised animals.

• **Grains, Bread, and Pastries:** All types of grains, pseudo-grains (like quinoa), and grain-based products such as bread and pasta are not allowed on the carnivore diet. These foods are high in carbohydrates, fiber, and anti-nutrients. They are also inflammatory, irritating to the gut, and may stimulate the immune system in certain individuals.

• **Nuts, Seeds, and Legumes:** Almonds, pecans, walnuts, peanuts, peas, flaxseeds, chia seeds, and all legumes are not allowed on the carnivore diet. These foods are high in carbohydrates, PUFAs (polyunsaturated fats), fiber, and anti-nutrients. They are also extremely difficult to digest and absorb by the body.

• **Anything That Isn't Animal-Based:** Candy, lab-grown meats, and meat alternatives like plant-based burgers are strictly excluded. The carnivore diet focuses solely on natural, whole animal-based foods and their byproducts, and eliminates all food items that come from other sources.

Carnivore Diet Spices

The decision to use herbs and spices in the carnivore diet depends on various factors such as individual context, goals, gut health status, and tolerance to specific foods. While a strict carnivore diet usually excludes herbs and spices, some individuals may choose to include them in trace amounts based on their personal preferences and sensitivities.

When considering the use of herbs and spices on the carnivore diet, it's important to be aware of their potential impact on inflammation and the presence of anti-nutrients. Anti-nutrients are compounds found in plants that can interfere with mineral absorption, irritate the gut, stimulate the immune system, and potentially lead to negative symptoms or exacerbate pre-existing chronic conditions.

Certain herbs and spices contain anti-nutrients such as oxalates and lectins, which may affect individuals who are sensitive to them. Oxalates, for example, may contribute to the formation of kidney stones and are associated with symptoms like fibromyalgia and thyroid dysfunction.

Herbs and spices with a high oxalate content include cinnamon, turmeric, black pepper, cumin seed, and allspice. On the other hand, herbs and spices with a low-oxalate content include garlic powder, white pepper, basil, cilantro, vanilla, mustard, thyme, red pepper flakes, paprika, cardamom, chilli powder, and cayenne pepper.

Lectins, another group of anti-nutrients, may cause symptoms such as bloating, gas, indigestion, and digestive disturbances, particularly in individuals who are sensitive to them. Nightshade vegetables, including tomatoes, potatoes, bell peppers, and eggplants, are known for their higher lectin content. Some spices that contain high levels of lectins include paprika, chili pepper flakes, cayenne pepper, cumin, peppermint, nutmeg, chilli powder, and curry powder. Conversely, low-lectin herbs and spices include onion powder, chives, fennel, parsley, basil, mint, cilantro, rosemary, sage, tarragon, thyme, oregano, ginger, and sage.

In general, when incorporating herbs and spices into the carnivore diet, it is recommended to choose those that are low in anti-nutrients and have a lower potential for inflammation. Leaves tend to be less inflammatory, while seeds are more likely to induce inflammation. Some examples of herbs and spices that are considered more suitable for the carnivore diet include basil, bay leaf, parsley, sage, vanilla bean, rosemary, thyme, dill, cilantro, chives, tarragon, oregano, ginger, and garlic.

It is important to ensure that any herbs or spices you choose are organic, free from added fillers, and fresh to maintain their quality, nutrient density, and minimize any risk of potential contamination. Additionally, it's crucial to listen to your body and pay attention to any adverse reactions or sensitivities you may experience when using herbs and spices.

Carnivore Diet Snacks

While the carnivore diet emphasizes the consumption of large, solid meals and discourages frequent snacking for optimal metabolic health and body composition, there may be occasions when you find yourself hungry but unable to have a complete, proper meal.

In such situations, having some carnivore-approved snacks available can help tide you over and provide a temporary source of energy until your next solid meal.

It's important to note that snacks should be consumed sparingly and not become a regular habit, especially if your goals include fat loss, autoimmune healing, or optimizing longevity.

Here are some carnivore-approved snacks that can be used when the need arises:

- **Pemmican:** Pemmican is a traditional snack made from dried and powdered meat mixed with rendered animal fat. It is a nutrient-dense option that provides quality protein and healthy fats. It can be a convenient and energy-rich snack.

- **Liver chips:** Liver chips are thinly sliced and dehydrated liver, offering a concentrated source of vitamins, minerals, trace elements, and other essential nutrients. They provide a flavorful and nutrient-packed snack option.

• **Bone broth:** Sipping on bone broth can be a satisfying snack, providing hydration, electrolytes, energy, and valuable amino acids derived from simmered animal bones and connective tissue. It can be a comforting and nourishing choice.

• **Hard-boiled eggs:** Hard-boiled eggs are a popular food item in most omnivorous diets, made by boiling eggs until the egg white and yolk solidify. They are known for their convenience, as they can be prepared in advance and stored in the refrigerator for several days. They offer a portable and protein-rich snack.

• **Mini meat pies:** Mini meat pies made with carnivore-approved ingredients, such as ground meat and animal fat, can be a convenient and satiating snack option. They can be prepared ahead of time and enjoyed on the go.

• **Beef jerky and meat sticks:** High-quality beef jerky and meat sticks made from minimal ingredients without added sugars or artificial additives can be a protein-packed, healthy snack on the carnivore diet. They offer a convenient and portable source of protein.

• **Liverwurst:** Liverwurst is a type of sausage that typically includes liver as one of the main ingredients, providing a concentrated source of nutrients like vitamins A, B12, and iron. It can be sliced and enjoyed as a flavorful and nutrient-dense snack.

- **Canned fish:** Canned fish such as sardines, mackerel, or salmon can be a convenient snack option, offering a good source of omega-3 fatty acids, protein, and various micronutrients. They provide a quick and nutritious snack.

- **Pork rinds:** Pork rinds, also known as pork skins or cracklings, are fried or roasted pieces of pig skin. They are crunchy and provide a low-carb, high-fat snack option. They can be enjoyed as a savory and satisfying snack.

It's important to choose snacks that align with the principles of the carnivore diet, meaning they primarily consist of animal-based ingredients and avoid additives, fillers, and added sugars. Additionally, when consuming these snacks, it's crucial to listen to your body's hunger and satiety cues to prevent overeating or using snacks as a substitute for proper meals.

Snacks on the carnivore diet should be seen as occasional and supplementary, and the focus should primarily be on consuming nutrient-dense, complete meals that fulfil your body's nutritional needs.

Ask Your Butcher For:

Beef

- Ribeye Steak

- New York Strip Steak
- T-bone Steak
- Ground Beef
- Short Ribs or Back Ribs
- Brisket
- Skirt Steak
- Tri-tip Steak
- Porterhouse Steak
- Chuck Roast
- Filet Mignon
- Strip Loin
- Tenderloin
- Flank Steak
- Roast Beef
- Beef Jerky
- Beef Sausage

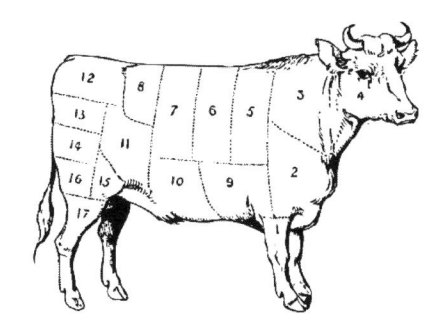

Chicken

- Rotisserie Chicken
- Chicken Wings
- Chicken Thighs
- Chicken Drumsticks
- Chicken Breast
- Chicken Ground Meat

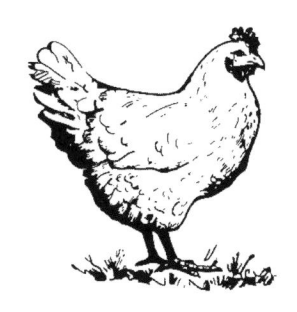

Pork

- Pork Ribs
- Pork Belly
- Pork Chops
- Pork Shoulder
- Pork Butt
- Pulled Pork
- Pork Sausage

Lamb

- Lamb Chops
- Lamb Shanks
- Lamb Shoulder
- Lamb Ground Meat
- Lamb Sausage

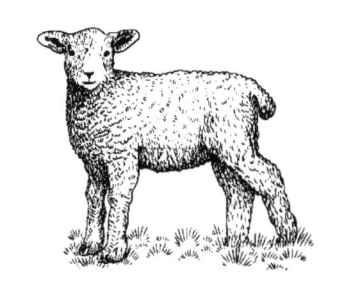

Bison

- Bison Ribeye
- Bison Striploin
- Bison Tenderloin
- Bison Sirloin
- Bison Ground Meat
- Bison Sausage

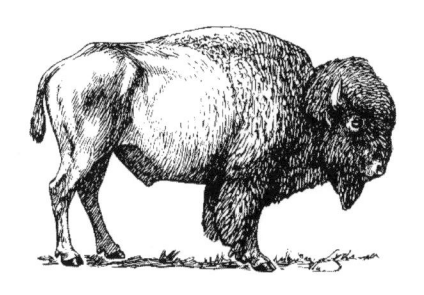

Organ Meats

- Liver
- Heart
- Oxtail
- Cheeks

- Tongue
- Brain
- Kidney
- Feet

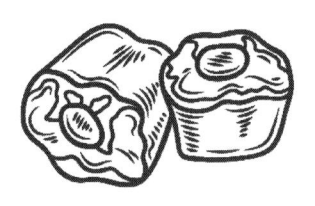

Ask Your Fishmonger For:

Fish & Seafood

- Salmon
- Shrimp
- Tuna
- Lobster
- Cod
- Crab

- Tilapia
- Scallops
- Mussels
- Trout
- Oysters
- Mahi-Mahi
- Clams
- Sardines
- Halibut
- Squid
- Anchovies
- Catfish
- Snapper
- Swordfish

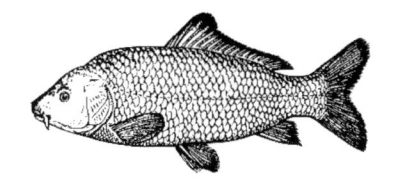

Look For the Following in the Organic Section:

Animal-Based Foods

- Chicken Eggs
- Duck Eggs
- Quail Eggs
- Goose Eggs
- Cow's Milk
- Goat's Milk
- Sheep's Milk
- Buffalo's Milk
- Camel's Milk
- Cheese
- Yogurt
- Butter
- Cream
- Kefir
- Bacon (soy-free, sugar-free, nitrate-free)

- Sausages

- Cured meats

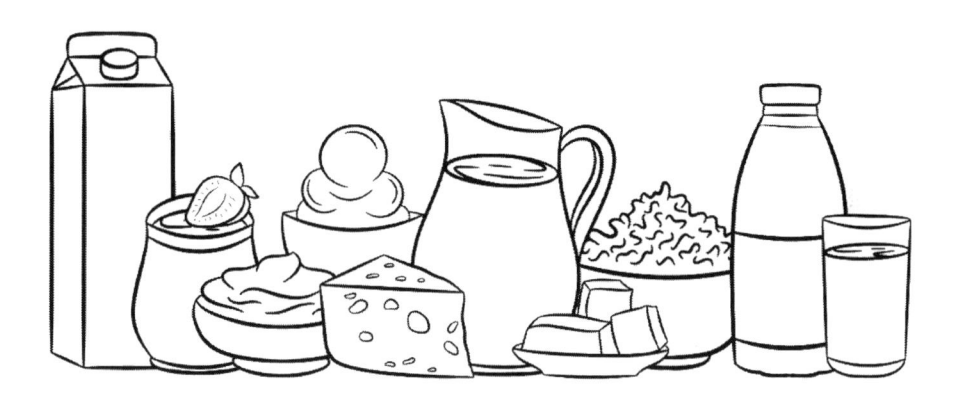

Do You Have to Eat Organ Meats?

Consuming organ meats is not a strict requirement in the carnivore diet, however, it is highly recommended for the following reasons:

• **Nutrient Density:** Organ meats are some of the most nutrient-dense foods on the planet. They are rich in essential vitamins, minerals, and trace elements, such as vitamin A, vitamin D, vitamin B12, iron, zinc, and copper. Including organ meats in the diet can help ensure an adequate intake of these important nutrients.

• **Unique Nutritional Profile:** Organ meats contain a unique nutritional profile compared to muscle meats. For example, liver is a concentrated source of vitamin A, folate, and iron, while heart is rich in coenzyme Q10 and other beneficial compounds. Incorporating a variety of organ meats can provide a broader spectrum of nutrients into your diet.

• **Bioavailability of Nutrients:** The nutrients found in organ meats are highly bioavailable, meaning they are easily absorbed and utilized by the body. This makes them an efficient source of essential nutrients that support various bodily functions, including energy production, immune function, and hormone synthesis.

• **Organ-Specific Health Benefits:** Organ meats have been associated with various organ-specific health benefits. For instance, liver is known for its role in supporting liver health and detoxification processes. Heart is believed to support cardiovascular health, and brain contains omega-3 fatty acids (especially DHA) that are beneficial for brain and cognitive function.

- **Traditional Dietary Practice:** Consuming organ meats has been a part of traditional dietary practices in many cultures throughout history. Our ancestors valued the whole animal and recognized the nutritional importance of consuming organ meats. Incorporating this ancestral wisdom into the carnivore diet can provide a more holistic and nutrient-rich approach to eating.

Palatability

While the carnivore diet allows for individual preferences and tolerances, incorporating organ meats can significantly enhance the nutritional value of the diet. If you find the taste of organ meats challenging, there are several strategies you can try to make them more palatable. These include:

- **Seasoning and Marinades:** Experiment with different seasonings, herbs, and spices to enhance the flavor of organ meats. Marinating them in acidic ingredients like lemon juice or vinegar can help tenderize the meat and reduce/neutralize any strong flavors.

- **Cooking Techniques:** Opt for cooking methods that can help mask the taste or texture of organ meats. For example, braising, slow cooking, or incorporating them into stews, soups, or casseroles can help blend their flavors with other ingredients.

- **Combining with Other Meats:** Mix organ meats with muscle meats or ground meats to balance out the flavors and textures. Combining them in meatloaf, meatballs, or burgers can make them more enjoyable.

- **Blending or Grinding:** If you're still hesitant about the taste, you can try blending or grinding organ meats and incorporating them into other dishes such as sauces, pâtés, or meat spreads. This way, you can still benefit from their nutritional value without the distinct taste.

- **Start with Milder Organ Meats:** Begin by trying milder-tasting organ meats like chicken liver or heart before moving on to stronger-flavored options like beef liver or kidneys. This can help ease you into the taste gradually.

- **Seek Expert Advice:** Consult with a professional chef, nutritionist, or registered dietitian who is knowledgeable about organ meats. They can provide guidance, tips, and recipes to make organ meats more enjoyable and appealing.

Keep in mind that taste preferences can vary, and it may take some time for you to develop a liking for organ meats. So, try to be open to experimenting with different cooking methods and recipes until you find a preparation that best suits your palate.

How to Choose Organ Meats

When seeking high-quality organ meats, you may consider the following factors:

• **Organic or pasture-raised:** Look for organ meats sourced from organically-raised or pasture-raised animals. These animals are typically raised in more natural and healthier environments, which can reduce the risk of exposure to toxins.

• **Grass-fed or grass-finished:** Opt for organ meats from animals that have been exclusively grass-fed or grass-finished. Grass-fed animals tend to have a superior nutrient profile compared to conventionally-raised animals, including organ meats.

• **Local and sustainable sources:** Consider sourcing organ meats from local farmers or suppliers who prioritize sustainable and ethical farming practices. Building a relationship with your local butcher or visiting farmer's markets can help you find high-quality options.

• **Third-party certifications:** Look for organ meats that carry certifications from reputable third-party organizations. Examples include: USDA Organic, Animal Welfare Approved, or Certified Humane. These certifications indicate adherence to specific standards of animal welfare and farming practices.

• **Transparent sourcing:** If possible, choose suppliers that provide transparency about their sourcing and farming practices. This could include information about the animals' diet, living conditions, and any additional certifications they hold.

• **Quality control:** Ensure that the supplier follows strict quality control measures, such as proper handling, storage, and transportation of the organ meats. This can help minimize the risk of contamination and maintain the nutrient density of the products.

Key Points

• Organ meats are extremely nutrient-dense and rich in essential vitamins, minerals, and trace elements. They provide important nutrients like vitamin A, vitamin D, vitamin B12, iron, zinc, and copper.

• Organ meats offer a unique nutritional profile compared to muscle meats. Liver is a concentrated source of vitamin A, folate, and iron, while heart contains coenzyme Q10 and other beneficial compounds.

• The nutrients in organ meats are highly bioavailable, easily absorbed and utilized by the body. They efficiently support energy production, immune function, and hormone synthesis.

• Organ meats have specific health benefits for different organs. Liver supports liver health and detoxification, heart promotes cardiovascular health, and brain contains omega-3 fatty acids beneficial for brain function.

• Consuming organ meats has been part of traditional dietary practices in many cultures. Our ancestors recognized the nutritional importance of organ meats for a holistic and nutrient-rich approach to eating.

Is Honey Carnivore?

Honey is an animal-based food product derived from insects within the animal kingdom, but the product itself, honey, doesn't contain any animal tissue or cells like dairy products, which are carnivore-friendly foods derived from animals. Thus, if you follow a strict, zero-carb carnivore diet, honey shouldn't be part of your diet.

On the opposite, if you are an athlete and physically active person, honey may comprise a great, gut-friendly, easy-to-digest, and nutritious source of carbs (fuel) and micronutrients for you. One of the main benefits of the carnivore diet is the elimination principle. A lot of people have food-related diseases or challenges, and by just eliminating plants, they see great relief. Thus, if you are a complete newbie to the carnivore diet, it is recommended to exclude honey altogether at the start and strategically introduce it at some point later.

Keep in mind that honey is very rich in carbohydrates and simple sugars, specifically glucose, fructose, and sucrose. There's nothing inherently wrong about carbohydrates, but some people shouldn't include them in their diet when trying to heal their metabolism and gut. As an example, if you suffer from SIBO or yeast overgrowth (e.g. *Candida* overgrowth), you should abstain from honey completely for some time.

In most cases, the inclusion of honey in the carnivore diet is a hot and debated topic of discussion. Some people support its inclusion, while others are completely against it.

How Honey Is Made?

Honey is produced by honey bees through a complex process. Bees collect nectar from flowers using their proboscis (a long, tubular mouthpart) and store it in a special honey stomach called the honey crop. Enzymes in the honey crop break down complex sugars in the nectar into simpler sugars. Once the bee returns to the hive, it regurgitates the partially processed nectar into the mouth of another bee, a process known as trophallaxis. This transfer of nectar between bees allows for further enzymatic breakdown and evaporation of excess moisture. Finally, the nectar is deposited into the honeycomb cells, where it is further dehydrated through the action of bees fanning their wings. The end result is honey.

Honey's color and flavor can vary based on the type of nectar collected by bees. Different flowers produce different nectar, resulting in variations in the characteristics of the honey. For instance, honey derived from orange blossom nectar will generally have a light color, while honey from avocado or wildflowers may exhibit a darker amber color.

Beekeepers typically harvest surplus honey from hives, which can amount to approximately 65 pounds per year. The honey is collected by removing the honeycomb frames and scraping off the beeswax caps that seal the honey within each cell. Once the caps are removed, the frames are placed in an extractor—a centrifuge that spins the frames, causing the honey to be expelled from the comb.

After extraction, the honey undergoes straining to eliminate any remaining wax or other particles. It's important to note that some beekeepers and bottlers may choose to heat the honey during this process, although raw (unheated) honey is generally considered superior from a nutritional and health standpoint.

Raw honey is minimally processed and retains its natural enzymes, antioxidants, and other beneficial compounds. Heating honey can potentially diminish some of its nutritional benefits. However, the decision to heat honey can vary among beekeepers and bottlers based on factors such as ease of processing or specific market preferences.

Ultimately, if you prefer to consume honey in its raw form, it's advisable to look for honey labeled as "raw" or "unheated" to ensure you are obtaining honey with its full nutritional potential and enzyme content.

Is Honey Healthier Than Sugar?

Honey can be considered a healthier alternative to table/processed sugar due to several reasons. While both honey and table sugar are sweeteners rich in simple sugars, there are notable differences in their composition and potential health benefits:

• **Nutrient content:** Honey contains small amounts of various nutrients, including minerals such as magnesium, potassium, zinc, and vitamins like vitamin B6 and vitamin C. These micronutrients provide some nutritional value compared to refined sugar, which lacks any significant nutrients.

• **Antioxidant properties:** Honey is known to possess antioxidant compounds such as flavonoids and phenolic acids. Antioxidants help protect the body against oxidative stress and have positive effects on overall health.

• **Glycemic index:** The glycemic index (GI) is a measure of how quickly a food raises blood sugar levels. Honey has a lower glycemic index compared to refined sugar, meaning it causes a slower and more gradual rise in blood sugar levels. However, it's important to note that honey still raises blood sugar and should be consumed in moderation, especially for individuals with diabetes or those who need to manage their blood sugar levels.

• **Potential antimicrobial properties:** Certain types of honey, such as Manuka honey, have been found to possess antimicrobial properties due to the presence of natural compounds like hydrogen peroxide and methylglyoxal. These properties make honey beneficial for wound healing and can help fight certain infections.

Despite these advantages over processed sugar, it's important to remember that honey is still a sweetener and should be consumed in moderation. Honey is a significant source of calories and can contribute to weight gain if consumed excessively. Additionally, honey is not recommended for infants under one year old due to the risk of infant botulism. Infant botulism is a rare but serious illness that can occur when infants consume honey contaminated with *Clostridium botulinum* spores. These spores can germinate in an infant's immature digestive system and produce toxins that can cause muscle weakness and other symptoms.

The digestive system of infants under one-year-old is not fully developed, and their immune system may not be able to effectively fight off the bacteria. As a precautionary measure, it is generally recommended to avoid giving honey to infants until they are at least one year old.

Some of the Healthiest People in the World Consume Large Amounts of Honey

Honey is the most energy-dense food found in nature. Thus, it is not surprising that where it exists honey is an important food for almost all hunter-gatherers. For example, raw honey and bee products in general have a very special role in the diet of the Hadza tribe. This African hunter-gatherer tribe that resides in central Tanzania is the most extensively studied nomadic group in the world. In the last couple of years, the Hadza tribe diet has gained extreme popularity among health circles due to its purported gut health and longevity-promoting benefits.

The Hadza tribe's diet consists of a combination of wild game animals, plant foods, fruits, tubers, and raw honey. During the dry season, when game animals are more abundant, meat consumption is higher. In contrast, during the wet season, when fruits and berries are more plentiful, honey consumption significantly increases.

Hadza women typically acquire honey that is close to the ground, while Hadza men climb tall baobab trees to raid the largest bee hives and acquire fresh, raw, sweet, liquid honey. Overall, honey accounts for a significant portion of the energy/calories in the Hadza diet, especially that of Hadza men.

Benefits of Raw Honey

Raw honey has been used as a folk remedy throughout history as it offers a variety of well-established health benefits and medical applications. Today, raw honey is even used in some hospitals as a treatment for open wounds (due to its antimicrobial benefits). Many of the health benefits of honey are specific to raw/unpasteurized honey.

Most of the honey we find in the grocery store is pasteurized. Heat kills unwanted bacteria and yeast, can improve color and texture, removes any crystallization, and extends honey's shelf life. At the same time, many of the beneficial nutrients and enzymes of honey get destroyed.

Raw honey, especially raw dark honey, is a great source of micronutrients and antioxidants. It contains an array of plant phytochemicals that act as free radical scavengers (antioxidants). Some types of raw honey have as many antioxidants as fruits and vegetables, which is quite fascinating. Antioxidants help protect our body from cell damage caused by free radicals, such as reactive oxygen species (ROS).

Free radicals promote aging and contribute to inflammation in our body, thus promoting the development of various chronic diseases, including cancer, neurodegenerative disorders, and heart disease. Research has shown that antioxidant compounds present in raw honey called polyphenols exert a protective effect against heart disease and other chronic inflammatory diseases. Raw honey also carries antibacterial and antifungal properties. Scientific studies have shown that raw honey can kill unwanted bacteria and fungi as it naturally contains hydrogen peroxide (H_2O_2), an antiseptic. Its potency as an antibacterial and antifungal agent varies depending on the type of honey. However, it's fair to say that raw honey is more than a folk remedy for these kinds of infections.

Concerning its macronutrient profile, a tablespoon (tbsp) of honey has about 64 total calories, 17 g of net carbs, 0.1 g of protein, 0 g of fat, and 0 g of fiber.

Some of the vitamins found in raw honey include ascorbic acid (vitamin C), pantothenic acid (vitamin B5), niacin (vitamin B3), and riboflavin (vitamin B2), along with minerals, such as calcium, copper, iron, magnesium, manganese, phosphorus, potassium, and zinc.

Raw Milk

Raw milk is a nutrient-rich liquid food produced by the mammary glands of mammals. It is the primary source of nutrition for young mammals. For those following the carnivore diet, raw milk can be considered an excellent source of animal-based carbohydrates, primarily in the form of lactose.

Raw milk is often preferred over pasteurized milk due to the nutrients, probiotics, and heat-sensitive enzymes it contains. Pasteurization is a process that involves heating milk to kill potential harmful bacteria, but it can also have a negative impact on the nutritional composition and bioavailability of the milk.

Raw milk encompasses a superior nutrient profile compared to pasteurized milk. It is a great source of vitamins, including vitamin A, vitamin D, vitamin B12, and various B vitamins. It also provides minerals and trace elements, such as calcium, magnesium, phosphorus, potassium, and zinc. Additionally, raw milk contains beneficial bacteria, enzymes, and other bioactive compounds that contribute to its widespread health benefits.

Probiotics are live microorganisms that can confer health benefits to the host when consumed in adequate amounts. Raw milk is known to contain a diverse array of beneficial bacteria, including species of *Lactobacillus* and *Bifidobacterium*, which are probiotics. These bacteria support gut health, metabolic health, and immune system function.

Enzymes are protein molecules that facilitate various biochemical reactions in the body. Raw milk contains heat-sensitive enzymes, such as lactase, lipase, and protease, which aid in the digestion and breakdown of lactose, fats, and proteins, respectively. The presence of these enzymes in raw milk enhances its digestibility, bioavailability, and nutrient absorption.

Raw Milk Benefits

People have been drinking raw milk straight from their cows, sheep, and goats for millennia. Raw milk has long been one of the most nutritionally complete foods in the human diet and an integral component of nearly every culture's cuisine. In today's super-sanitized, germophobic, and technologically advanced world, raw milk is irrationally demonized for various reasons.

Dairy, especially cow dairy, can indeed be problematic for a lot of people. However, dairy derived from goats, sheep, or buffalo is much more gut- and immune-friendly due to the chemical structure of casein (milk protein) it contains. On top of that, many individuals who normally are lactose intolerant often find that they can tolerate raw milk just fine. These people actually have a pasteurization intolerance, not a dairy intolerance.

A reason that this happens is that raw milk naturally contains the enzyme lactase and specific probiotic species, like *Lactococcus, Lactobacillus, Leuconostoc, Streptococcus*, and *Enterococcus* which break down lactose, a disaccharide found in milk, into galactose and glucose, which are digestible, simple sugars.

Raw milk has for decades been well-regarded in health circles due to its unique health-promoting benefits:

• Raw milk provides readily available nutritional elements our body needs for repair and regeneration, including easily assimilable proteins and fats in their whole, unprocessed, unadulterated form.

• The fatty acids in raw milk nourish the brain and intestinal lining, and upregulate mitochondrial function, thus increasing cellular energy output. Mitochondria are membrane-bound cell organelles that generate most of the chemical energy needed to power the cell's biochemical reactions.

• Raw milk contains the enzyme phosphatase and other crucial enzymes necessary for the complete absorption of calcium, which are not present in pasteurized milk. That's why some research papers (falsely) link dairy consumption with the onset, rather than the prevention, of osteoporosis.

• Naturally occurring beneficial bacteria (probiotics) in raw milk carry amazing benefits for gut, immune, metabolic, and digestive health.

• Raw milk is a perfect source of unheated, unoxidized cholesterol, fatty acids, and non-denatured proteins. Protein denaturing or protein denaturation is a change in the chemical structure of protein that occurs due to chemical effects. The most common source of protein denaturing is heat application, as happens in pasteurization and cooking.

• Raw milk is nature's perfect electrolyte drink. It contains large amounts of organic minerals and trace elements, which nourish the body's organs and glands, provide intracellular hydration, and optimize brain function and performance.

• Colostrum (first mammal's milk after birth), but raw milk as well, contain immunoglobulins/antibodies, and complement factors that upregulate immune function and provide major antimicrobial benefits against a wide range of pathogens.

• People with bone-related conditions, like bone spurs, osteopenia, and osteoporosis, notice their condition significantly improving or even completely disappearing after a few months of daily ingestion of fresh, raw milk.

Where to Find Raw Milk?

Raw milk is not the easiest product to obtain, since its distribution in many countries and U.S. states is illegal. Many food and drug administrations around the world state that raw milk is particularly fertile for germs because it is unpasteurized, therefore not safe for human consumption.

This may apply to poor quality raw milk coming from unsanitary, industrially-raised animals. Raw milk sourced from healthy and happy ruminants naturally contains anti-microbial enzymes and probiotics that antagonize and inhibit pathogenic bacteria proliferation, such as *Salmonella*, *E. coli*, *Listeria*, *Campylobacter*, and others that cause foodborne illness, also known as food poisoning.

A good way to access raw milk (if the legal route is not an option), is by asking local farmers whether they might sell you some directly. Realmilk.com is a great online resource for learning about the safety and health benefits of raw milk. Realmilk.com also includes a searchable database of farmers that sell raw milk around the world.

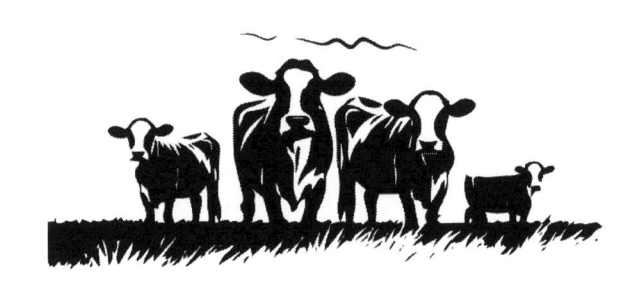

Carnivore Diet Shopping List

To successfully follow the carnivore diet, it's important to have a well-curated shopping list available to you. You may use the following carnivore diet shopping list as your starting guide:

Groceries

- Meat (all kinds)
- Eggs (pastured-raised)
- Dairy (preferably low-carb options, such as hard cheeses, butter, and cream)
- Animal fats for cooking (i.e. tallow, ghee, lard, or duck fat)
- Organ Meats
- Sparkling water
- Pink Himalayan salt or sea salt
- Electrolytes (for hydration, energy, and performance)
- Chicken or beef bone broth (for hydration, gut, immune, and connective tissue health)
- Spices, seasoning
- Coffee and tea (for the initial transition phase)

Equipment

- Air fryer (great, easy, and fast way to cook your meats)
- Vacuum sealer (allows you to keep meat fresh for a long time without the need to freeze it)
- Steak knife
- Knife sharpener
- Cutting board
- Cast iron skillet
- Frywall
- Dehydrator for jerky
- Grill
- Sous vide
- Pressure cooker
- Slow Cooker
- Instant Pot

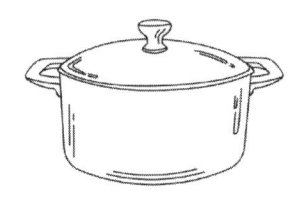

Carnivore Diet Meal Ideas

Breakfasts

Classic Combo

Start your day with a satisfying and nourishing breakfast by enjoying a classic combination of whole eggs and bacon. This timeless duo not only provides a burst of flavor but also offers a powerhouse of essential nutrients and protein to fuel your day.

Eggs, known for their versatility and nutritional value, are a staple in many diets, including the carnivore diet. They are an excellent source of high-quality protein, containing all nine essential amino acids that your body needs for various functions, including muscle repair and growth. Eggs are also rich in essential vitamins and minerals such as vitamin B12, vitamin D, selenium, and choline, which are important for maintaining optimal health and wellness.

Bacon, with its irresistible aroma and savory taste, adds a delicious element to the breakfast plate. It is a popular choice among carnivore enthusiasts due to its high-fat content and rich flavor. Bacon is primarily composed of fat, providing a good source of energy for the body. It also contains protein, vitamins B1, B3, B6, and minerals like zinc and selenium.

When combined, eggs and bacon create a satisfying and balanced breakfast that fuels your body with essential nutrients. The protein from the eggs helps promote satiety and supports muscle repair and growth, while the fat from the bacon provides a source of energy and adds a savory component to the meal.

To prepare this classic combo, simply cook your eggs to your preferred style, whether it's scrambled, fried, poached, or boiled. Pair the eggs with crispy, cooked bacon strips, allowing the flavors to mingle and create a harmonious blend of textures and tastes. You can also experiment with different cooking techniques, such as baking the bacon in the oven or adding herbs and spices to the eggs for additional flavor variations.

Not only does this breakfast option satisfy your taste buds, but it also provides a substantial amount of protein, healthy fats, vitamins, and minerals to kickstart your day. Remember to source high-quality eggs and bacon from pastured or organic sources whenever possible to ensure optimal nutrient content and to support animal welfare practices.

Gourmet Twist

Elevate your breakfast experience with a gourmet twist by preparing eggs in grass-fed butter and enhancing them with the delightful flavors of ham and cheese. This culinary creation not only promises a symphony of tastes but also offers a nourishing and low-carb way to begin your day.

Grass-fed butter, derived from the milk of cows that graze on natural grass pastures, boasts a rich and creamy texture that adds a luxurious touch to any dish. It is prized for its higher content of beneficial nutrients like omega-3 fatty acids, conjugated linoleic acid (CLA), and fat-soluble vitamins, such as vitamin A, vitamin E, and vitamin K2. Incorporating grass-fed butter into your breakfast not only enhances the flavor but also contributes to a well-rounded nutritional profile.

Eggs, the versatile and nutrient-packed stars of this dish, provide an excellent source of protein, vitamins, minerals, and trace elements. When cooked in grass-fed butter, they take on a velvety texture and a subtly buttery taste that elevates their flavor. Eggs are not only rich in high-quality protein but also provide essential nutrients like choline, which supports brain function, and lutein and zeaxanthin, which promote eye health. Additionally, they contain vitamins such as vitamin B12, vitamin D, and vitamin E, as well as minerals like selenium and iron.

To further enhance this gourmet breakfast, the addition of ham and cheese introduces layers of savory goodness. Ham, with its smoky and salty notes, pairs perfectly with the eggs and adds depth to the overall flavor profile. It is a good source of protein and contains essential vitamins and minerals, including vitamin B6, vitamin B12, zinc, and iron. When selecting ham, opt for minimally processed options without added sugars or artificial ingredients.

Cheese, with its wide array of flavors and textures, contributes a creamy and indulgent element to the dish. Choose from an assortment of cheese varieties, such as cheddar, Swiss, or Gouda, based on your personal preferences. Cheese offers a significant source of protein, calcium, and other essential nutrients. It also adds a satisfying richness to the breakfast, making it a delightful and satiating choice.

To prepare this gourmet twist, start by melting grass-fed butter in a skillet over medium heat. Crack the eggs into the skillet and cook them to your desired style, whether it's sunny-side-up, over-easy, or scrambled. As the eggs cook, the butter imparts a luscious flavor and helps create a beautifully golden and tender texture.

Once the eggs are cooked, layer thin slices of ham over the eggs, allowing their smoky essence to infuse into the dish. Sprinkle grated or sliced cheese over the ham and eggs, allowing it to melt slightly and form a delectable, gooey layer.

As you savor each bite of this gourmet breakfast, you'll experience the harmonious blend of the buttery eggs, the savory ham, and the creamy cheese. The combination of these flavors creates a breakfast sensation that satisfies your taste buds while providing a wealth of essential nutrients, including protein, healthy fats, vitamins, and minerals.

Indulge in this gourmet twist on breakfast, knowing that you're starting your day with a nourishing and low-carb option that delights your senses and supports your health and well-being.

Seafood Boost

Give your breakfast a nutrient-rich boost by combining pasture-raised eggs with the omega-3 fatty acid powerhouse, sardines. This unique pairing not only adds a delicious twist to your morning meal but also provides a multitude of health benefits.

Pasture-raised eggs come from hens that have access to outdoor areas where they can forage on a natural diet rich in insects, seeds, and plants. These eggs are known to have a more favorable nutritional profile compared to conventional eggs. They contain higher levels of omega-3 fatty acids, including eicosapentaenoic acid (EPA) and docosahexaenoic acid (DHA), which are essential for brain health, cardiovascular function, and reducing inflammation in the body. Pasture-raised eggs also tend to have higher levels of fat-soluble vitamins, such as vitamin A, vitamin E, and vitamin D.

Sardines, small fatty fish packed with nutrients, are a remarkable addition to this breakfast combination. They are an excellent source of omega-3 fatty acids, particularly EPA and DHA, which provide numerous health benefits. Omega-3 fatty acids play a crucial role in reducing inflammation, supporting brain health, improving heart health, and promoting healthy skin. Sardines are also a great source of high-quality protein, which is essential for muscle growth, repair, and overall body function. Additionally, they contain an array of important vitamins and minerals, including vitamin D, vitamin B12, calcium, selenium, and phosphorus.

To prepare this seafood-boosted breakfast, start by cooking your pasture-raised eggs according to your preference, whether it's scrambled, poached, or sunny-side-up. While the eggs cook, open a can of high-quality sardines packed in water or olive oil. Drain any excess liquid and gently place the sardines on a plate alongside the eggs.

When you take a bite of the rich and creamy eggs combined with the flavorful sardines, you'll experience a symphony of flavors and textures. The eggs provide a velvety backdrop, while the sardines offer a savory and slightly briny taste. This combination not only tantalizes your taste buds but also provides a balanced and complete source of protein, essential fatty acids, and a host of vitamins and minerals.

By incorporating this seafood boost into your breakfast routine, you're nourishing your body with a powerful combination of nutrients that support brain function, heart health, and overall well-being. The omega-3 fatty acids from the sardines and the protein from the pasture-raised eggs make this a true powerhouse meal, providing you with sustained energy and essential building blocks for optimal health.

Shrimp Delight

Indulge in a delectable and nutritious breakfast by combining the delicate flavors of shrimp with eggs and a touch of organic heavy cream. This delightful meal not only satisfies your taste buds but also provides a creamy, protein-rich start to your day that will keep you energized and satisfied.

Shrimp, known for their succulent taste and tender texture, are an excellent addition to your breakfast routine. They are a low-calorie, low-fat source of high-quality protein, making them an ideal choice for those seeking a satisfying and nutrient-dense meal. Shrimp also contain an impressive array of vitamins and minerals, including vitamin B12, vitamin D, selenium, and iodine. These nutrients play crucial roles in supporting overall health, including brain function, immune system function, and thyroid health.

To create this shrimp delight, begin by heating a non-stick skillet over medium heat. Add a small amount of cooking oil or grass-fed butter and allow it to melt. Once the skillet is hot, add the shrimp and cook them until they turn pink and opaque, typically for about 2-3 minutes per side. Remove the cooked shrimp from the skillet and set them aside.

In a separate bowl, whisk together the eggs and a splash of organic heavy cream. The addition of heavy cream lends a rich and velvety texture to the eggs, making them even more indulgent. Pour the egg mixture into the same skillet and cook them over medium heat, stirring gently until they reach your desired level of doneness. The result is a creamy and fluffy bed of scrambled eggs.

Next, gently fold in the cooked shrimp, allowing their flavors to blend harmoniously with the eggs. The combination of the mild sweetness of the shrimp and the creamy eggs creates a delightful symphony of flavors that will tantalize your taste buds.

Not only does this shrimp delight breakfast offer a delightful eating experience, but it also provides a powerful nutritional punch. The eggs contribute to the meal's protein content, supporting muscle growth, repair, and satiety. The shrimp not only add more protein but also supply essential nutrients like iodine, which plays a vital role in thyroid function. Additionally, the organic heavy cream adds a touch of healthy fats and creaminess, contributing to a balanced macronutrient profile.

By starting your day with this shrimp delight breakfast, you're treating yourself to a nutritious and satisfying meal that fuels your body with essential nutrients. The combination of shrimp, eggs, and organic heavy cream offers a harmonious blend of flavors and textures, creating a breakfast experience that is both delightful and nourishing.

Salmon and Sausage

Elevate your breakfast experience by savoring the richness of salmon paired with flavorful turkey sausage and eggs. This tantalizing combination not only delivers a delicious blend of flavors but also offers a diverse mix of proteins and healthy fats to power your morning.

Salmon, known for its vibrant pink color and buttery texture, is a nutritional powerhouse. Packed with omega-3 fatty acids, high-quality protein, and essential vitamins and minerals, salmon is a superb addition to any meal, especially breakfast. Omega-3 fatty acids play a crucial role in supporting heart health, brain function, and reducing inflammation in the body. The protein content in salmon helps promote muscle growth, repair, and satiety, making it an excellent choice for those seeking a satisfying and nourishing breakfast.

Turkey sausage, on the other hand, adds a savory and slightly spicy element to this breakfast ensemble. Made from lean turkey meat, it provides a leaner alternative to traditional pork sausage while still delivering an abundance of flavor and nutrients. Turkey sausage offers a good source of protein and supplies essential nutrients such as iron, zinc, and B vitamins, which are vital for energy production and overall well-being.

To prepare this delightful breakfast, start by cooking the turkey sausage in a skillet over medium heat. Allow it to brown and cook thoroughly, breaking it up into crumbles as it cooks. Once the turkey sausage is cooked, remove it from the skillet and set it aside.

In the same skillet, add a small amount of cooking oil or grass-fed butter and heat it over medium heat. Place the salmon fillets in the skillet, skin-side down, and cook them for a few minutes until they develop a golden crust. Flip the fillets and continue cooking until they are cooked through and flake easily with a fork. Remove the salmon from the skillet and set it aside.

In a separate bowl, whisk together the eggs until they are well-beaten. Pour the beaten eggs into the skillet and cook them over medium heat, stirring gently until they reach your desired level of doneness. The eggs should be fluffy and cooked to perfection.

To assemble your breakfast plate, arrange the cooked turkey sausage, flaked salmon, and scrambled eggs together. The combination of savory turkey sausage, the rich flavors of salmon, and the fluffy scrambled eggs creates a symphony of tastes and textures that will awaken your senses.

Not only does this breakfast provide a satisfying culinary experience, but it also offers a wide range of nutritional benefits. The omega-3 fatty acids from the salmon, coupled with the high-quality protein from both the salmon and turkey sausage, make this meal an excellent source of essential nutrients. These nutrients support brain health, heart health, muscle growth, and overall well-being.

By indulging in this salmon and sausage breakfast, you're treating yourself to a delightful and nourishing start to the day. The combination of flavorful salmon, savory turkey sausage, and perfectly scrambled eggs ensures that your morning is filled with a balance of proteins and healthy fats, providing sustained energy and satiety.

Chicken and Sausage

Kickstart your day with a hearty and protein-packed breakfast by combining eggs, tender chicken, and flavorful sausage. This delicious and satisfying meal provides a nutritious boost that will keep you feeling full, energized, and ready to tackle your morning activities.

Chicken, known for its versatility and lean protein content, offers a range of health benefits. It is a great source of high-quality protein, essential amino acids, and important vitamins and minerals. Protein is essential for muscle repair, growth, and overall maintenance of the body's tissues. It also plays a vital role in supporting satiety and regulating blood sugar levels, helping to control cravings and promote a balanced appetite.

Sausage, with its savory flavors and variety of seasonings, adds a delicious twist to this breakfast combination. Opting for quality sausage made from lean meats and minimal additives ensures a healthier option. Sausage provides additional protein, essential fats, and a burst of flavors that enhance the overall taste of the dish.

To prepare this satisfying breakfast, begin by cooking the sausage in a skillet over medium heat. Allow it to brown and cook thoroughly, breaking it into smaller pieces as it cooks. Once the sausage is cooked to perfection, transfer it to a plate lined with paper towels to absorb any excess grease.

Next, in the same skillet, add a small amount of cooking oil or grass-fed butter and heat it over medium heat. Add the diced chicken to the skillet, seasoned with your preferred herbs and spices, and cook until it is cooked through and no longer pink in the center. The chicken will contribute a tender and flavorful protein source to the breakfast ensemble.

While the chicken is cooking, whisk the eggs in a bowl until they are well-beaten. Once the chicken is cooked, pour the beaten eggs into the skillet with the chicken and cook them over medium heat. Stir gently until the eggs are scrambled to your desired consistency. The combination of chicken, sausage, and eggs will create a satisfying and protein-rich base for your breakfast.

To serve, plate the scrambled eggs alongside the cooked chicken and sausage, allowing the flavors to mingle and complement each other. The hearty combination of chicken and sausage brings a delightful variety of textures and flavors, making each bite a delicious experience.

Not only does this breakfast dish satisfy your taste buds, but it also provides essential nutrients to fuel your day. The protein from the chicken and sausage supports muscle repair and growth, while the eggs provide additional protein, vitamins, and minerals. This combination of proteins will help you feel satiated, regulate your blood sugar levels, and provide a sustained source of energy throughout the morning.

By enjoying this chicken and sausage breakfast, you're not only treating yourself to a flavorful and satisfying meal, but you're also giving your body the nutrients it needs to thrive. So, indulge in this protein-packed breakfast, and enjoy the benefits of feeling nourished, energized, and ready to conquer your day.

Liver Boost

Elevate the nutritional value of your breakfast by incorporating the powerhouse organ meat known as liver. Adding a small piece of liver to your breakfast eggs not only introduces a unique and rich flavor but also provides a multitude of health benefits that make it a valuable addition to your carnivore diet.

Liver, often referred to as nature's multivitamin, is packed with essential nutrients that are vital for overall health and well-being. It is an abundant source of various B vitamins, including vitamin B12, vitamin B6, riboflavin (vitamin B2), and folate (vitamin B9). These B vitamins play crucial roles in energy production, brain function, red blood cell formation, and the metabolism of amino acids and fatty acids.

In addition to B vitamins, liver is a rich source of vitamin A, which is essential for maintaining healthy vision, supporting immune function, and promoting cell growth and differentiation. Liver also contains significant amounts of vitamin D, vitamin E, and vitamin K, all of which contribute to various aspects of health, including bone health, antioxidant protection, and blood clotting regulation.

Minerals such as iron, zinc, copper, selenium, and manganese are also found in abundance in liver. Iron is critical for the production of hemoglobin and the transportation of oxygen throughout the body. Zinc is involved in numerous enzymatic reactions, immune system function, and wound healing. Copper is essential for collagen production, iron metabolism, and antioxidant defence. Selenium acts as a potent antioxidant, while manganese is involved in bone formation and carbohydrate metabolism.

Furthermore, liver is a concentrated source of highly bioavailable protein, containing all the essential amino acids required for various physiological functions. The amino acids found in liver contribute to muscle growth, tissue repair, hormone synthesis, and enzyme production.

To incorporate liver into your breakfast, start by selecting a high-quality, grass-fed or pasture-raised liver from a reputable source. Slice a small piece of liver, ensuring it is fresh and free from any visible abnormalities. Heat a skillet over medium heat and add a small amount of cooking fat, such as grass-fed butter or ghee. Place the liver slices in the skillet and cook them for a few minutes on each side until they are cooked through but still tender.

While the liver is cooking, prepare your eggs according to your preference, whether scrambled, poached, or fried. Once the liver is cooked, remove it from the skillet and set it aside. Combine the cooked liver with your eggs, allowing the flavors to meld together.

By incorporating liver into your breakfast, you are infusing your meal with an array of essential nutrients that support optimal health and vitality. The unique flavors and textures of liver add depth and richness to your breakfast eggs, making each bite a nourishing experience.

Beef Burger Power

Indulge in a breakfast that combines the mouthwatering flavors of a juicy beef burger patty with the creamy goodness of cheese. This hearty meal not only satisfies your taste buds but also provides a wealth of nutrients and energy to fuel your day.

Choosing a high-quality beef burger patty is key to maximizing the nutritional benefits of this breakfast option. Opt for grass-fed or pasture-raised beef, as these sources tend to have a higher content of beneficial nutrients compared to conventionally-raised beef. Grass-fed beef is known to contain higher levels of omega-3 fatty acids, conjugated linoleic acid (CLA), and antioxidant vitamins, such as vitamin E.

Beef is an excellent source of complete protein, providing all the essential amino acids your body needs for muscle growth, repair, and maintenance. Protein is also essential for supporting immune function, enzyme production, and hormone synthesis. Additionally, beef is rich in iron, zinc, selenium, and B vitamins, including vitamin B12, which is vital for red blood cell production and neurological health.

When selecting the cheese for your beef burger patty, consider opting for high-quality, full-fat varieties. Cheese is a good source of calcium, phosphorus, and vitamin A. It also contains protein, healthy fats, and fat-soluble vitamins, like vitamin K2, which plays a role in bone health and calcium metabolism.

To prepare your beef burger patty, start with a high-quality ground beef that is ideally 80% lean and 20% fat for optimal flavor and juiciness. Season the meat with your preferred seasonings such as salt, pepper, garlic powder, or any herbs and spices of your choice. Shape the ground beef into patties of your desired thickness.

Cook the beef burger patty to your preferred level of doneness, whether rare, medium-rare, medium, or well-done. You can grill it on a barbecue, cook it on a stovetop griddle, or even broil it in the oven. Make sure to cook it thoroughly to ensure food safety.

When the burger patty is almost done, top it with a slice of your favorite cheese, such as cheddar, Swiss, or pepper jack. Allow the cheese to melt and become slightly gooey, adding a luscious and flavorful element to your burger.

To enhance the nutritional value of your breakfast, consider adding additional toppings or condiments that align with your carnivore diet preferences. Some options could include bacon or fried eggs. These additions can further enhance the flavor and nutrient profile of your beef burger breakfast.

Enjoy your beef burger patty topped with cheese as a savory and satisfying breakfast option. The combination of high-quality beef and cheese not only delivers a burst of deliciousness but also provides a wealth of essential nutrients to kick-start your day with energy and satisfaction. Remember to choose grass-fed or pasture-raised beef and opt for full-fat, high-quality cheese to maximize the nutritional benefits of this indulgent breakfast.

Pork Indulgence

Treat yourself to a hearty and flavorful breakfast by combining the succulent flavors of pork sausage and bacon. This indulgent combination not only satisfies your taste buds but also provides a wealth of quality protein, healthy fats, and essential nutrients to fuel your morning.

Pork sausage and bacon are both excellent sources of protein, which is essential for building and repairing tissues, supporting immune function, and producing enzymes and hormones. Protein-rich foods help keep you feeling full and satisfied, reducing cravings and supporting healthy weight management and metabolic health.

When selecting pork sausage and bacon for your breakfast, opt for high-quality, minimally-processed options. Look for products made from pasture-raised or organic pork, as these sources tend to have a superior nutritional profile. Pasture-raised pork is known to contain higher levels of omega-3 fatty acids, vitamin D, and antioxidant nutrients (i.e. selenium, zinc, vitamin E), compared to conventionally-raised pork.

Pork sausage is typically seasoned with a variety of herbs and spices, enhancing its flavor and providing additional health benefits. Some sausage varieties may include ingredients like fennel seeds, sage, thyme, or garlic, which not only add delicious taste but also offer antioxidant and anti-inflammatory benefits.

Bacon, on the other hand, is renowned for its rich, smoky flavor and crispy texture. It is important to note that not all bacon products are created equal. Opt for bacon that is free from added sugars, nitrates, and artificial additives. Look for brands that use traditional curing methods or choose uncured bacon options that use natural ingredients, like celery powder, for preservation.

Pork sausage and bacon are also excellent sources of healthy fats. While pork fat contains a mix of saturated and monounsaturated fats, it also provides beneficial omega-3 and omega-6 fatty acids. These fats play important roles in brain health, hormone production, and reducing inflammation in the body.

Moreover, pork products like sausage and bacon contain fat-soluble vitamins, such as vitamin A, vitamin D, vitamin E, and vitamin K2. These vitamins are crucial for various bodily functions, including immune system support, bone health, vision, and blood clotting.

To enjoy the pork indulgence breakfast, you can cook the pork sausage and bacon in a skillet until they are browned and cooked through. Serve them alongside eggs prepared to your liking, whether scrambled, fried, or poached. This combination of protein-rich pork sausage, crispy bacon, and eggs provides a balanced and satisfying breakfast option.

Steak Perfection

Elevate your breakfast experience with a small, perfectly cooked beef steak seasoned with a touch of sea salt. This indulgent morning meal not only delights your taste buds but also offers a wealth of essential nutrients and flavors that are sure to kickstart your day on a high note.

When choosing a beef steak for your breakfast, opt for high-quality cuts such as ribeye, tenderloin, or sirloin.

These cuts tend to be tender, juicy, and rich in flavor. Selecting grass-fed or pasture-raised beef can further enhance the nutritional profile of your steak, as it is known to have higher levels of beneficial omega-3 fatty acids and antioxidants.

Beef is an excellent source of high-quality protein, containing all the essential amino acids your body needs for growth, repair, and maintenance of tissues. Protein is also essential for the production of enzymes, hormones, and antibodies, as well as supporting healthy muscle function.

In addition to protein, beef steak provides an array of essential vitamins and minerals. It is a rich source of B vitamins, including vitamin B12, which is necessary for proper brain function and the production of red blood cells. It also contains important minerals, like iron, zinc, and selenium, which play key roles in immune function, metabolism, and antioxidant defence.

When cooking your beef steak, aim for the desired level of doneness that suits your preferences. Whether you prefer a rare, medium-rare, or well-done steak, ensure proper cooking temperatures are reached to ensure food safety. Season your steak with a sprinkle of sea salt, which not only enhances the flavor but also adds a touch of minerals to your meal.

Seafood Twist

Awaken your taste buds and add a touch of elegance to your morning routine with a delightful seafood twist in your breakfast. Combine the delicate flavors of trout, a freshwater fish rich in omega-3 fatty acids, with tender shreds of chicken for a breakfast option that is both light and satisfying.

Trout, known for its mild and slightly nutty flavor, is a versatile fish that provides an abundance of essential nutrients. It is an excellent source of high-quality protein, which is essential for muscle repair, growth, and overall body function. Additionally, trout is rich in omega-3 fatty acids, particularly eicosapentaenoic acid (EPA) and docosahexaenoic acid (DHA), which are known for their anti-inflammatory properties and their role in supporting heart health and brain function.

Shredded chicken, on the other hand, adds a complementary protein component to the dish. Chicken is a lean source of protein that offers a complete amino acid profile necessary for the synthesis and repair of body tissues. It is also a good source of B vitamins, such as niacin and vitamin B6, which are involved in energy metabolism and nervous system function.

To prepare this seafood twist breakfast, start by gently cooking the trout until it is tender and flakes easily with a fork. Season it with a sprinkle of sea salt and your favorite herbs and spices to enhance its natural flavors. Meanwhile, cook and shred the chicken, ensuring it is thoroughly cooked and free from any pinkness in the center.

To serve, arrange the cooked trout and shredded chicken on a plate, creating an appealing and colorful presentation. You may also add a squeeze of lemon juice to brighten the flavors and provide a refreshing tang.

Snacks

Jerky Delights

Indulge in the savory goodness of jerky for a satisfying and protein-packed snack. Choose from an array of options such as beef, bison, turkey, or salmon jerky, all of which offer unique flavors and textures to suit your taste preferences. When selecting jerky, it's important to opt for soy-free, sugar-free, and nitrate-free varieties to ensure a clean and carnivore-friendly snack that aligns with the principles of the carnivore diet.

Jerky is a dehydrated meat product that has been enjoyed for centuries due to its portability, long shelf life, and concentrated protein content. It is made by marinating and drying strips of lean meat, resulting in a flavorful and chewy snack that can be conveniently carried and enjoyed on-the-go.

Beef jerky, one of the most popular choices, is typically made from high-quality cuts of lean beef. It is rich in protein, essential amino acids, and various vitamins and minerals, such as iron, zinc, and B vitamins. The drying process helps preserve the nutrients, making beef jerky a concentrated source of nourishment.

Turkey jerky offers a leaner alternative with a milder flavor. It is made from lean cuts of turkey meat, which provides ample protein and is often lower in fat compared to beef. Turkey jerky is also a good source of essential minerals like iron, phosphorus, and selenium, as well as B vitamins that support energy production and overall well-being.

For seafood enthusiasts, salmon jerky offers a unique and omega-3 fatty acid-rich option. Salmon is renowned for its impressive content of EPA and DHA, omega-3 fatty acids that promote heart health, brain function, and reduced inflammation in the body. Salmon jerky provides a convenient way to incorporate these beneficial fatty acids into your diet while enjoying a flavorful snack.

When selecting jerky, be sure to read the ingredient list and opt for varieties that are free from soy, added sugars, nitrates, and other preservatives. These additives do not align with the carnivore diet, which emphasizes whole, unprocessed foods. Look for brands that use natural seasonings and spices to enhance the flavor of the jerky without compromising its nutritional integrity.

Jerky can be enjoyed as a standalone snack or paired with other carnivore-friendly options, like cheese or hard-boiled eggs, for a more substantial meal. Its portability makes it an excellent choice for busy days, outdoor activities, or as a quick and convenient source of protein during travel.

Remember to listen to your body's hunger and fullness cues and consume jerky in moderation as a snack. While it is a convenient and nutrient-dense option, it's important to incorporate a variety of animal-based foods to ensure you cover your body's nutritional needs.

Crunchy Pork Rinds

Indulge in the satisfying crunch of pork rinds, a beloved snack among carnivores and those following a keto diet. These light and crispy treats are made from the skin of pigs that has been fried or roasted, resulting in a delightful snack that is rich in flavor and texture.

Pork rinds, also known as pork skins or chicharrones, have gained popularity for their low-carb and high-fat profile, making them a suitable choice for individuals seeking a satisfying snack while adhering to a carnivore or ketogenic lifestyle. While traditionally enjoyed as a snack, pork rinds can also be used as a versatile ingredient in various recipes.

One of the significant advantages of pork rinds is their protein content. They provide a substantial amount of high-quality protein, which is essential for tissue repair, muscle maintenance, and overall body function. Protein is also known to induce satiety, making pork rinds a satisfying snack option that can help curb hunger between meals.

Pork rinds are also rich in healthy fats. While they are fried, the fat content primarily comes from the natural fat present in the pork skin itself. These fats can provide a source of energy, support hormone production, and aid in the absorption of fat-soluble vitamins.

Speaking of vitamins, pork rinds contain several fat-soluble vitamins, including vitamin A, vitamin E, and vitamin D. These vitamins play important roles in various bodily functions, such as promoting healthy vision, supporting immune function, and aiding in calcium absorption for strong bones.

Additionally, pork rinds are naturally carb-free, making them a suitable option for individuals following a low-carb or ketogenic diet. They are a satisfying alternative to traditional carb-laden snacks like chips or crackers, allowing you to enjoy a crunchy and flavorful treat without the added carbohydrates.

When selecting pork rinds, it's important to choose high-quality options that are free from added preservatives, artificial flavors, or excessive seasoning. Opt for brands that use minimal ingredients and adhere to a clean and unprocessed approach.

While pork rinds can be enjoyed on their own as a snack, they can also be used creatively in recipes. Crushed pork rinds can be used as a low-carb breading for meat or poultry, providing a crispy coating without the need for traditional bread crumbs. They can also be added to salads or used as a crunchy topping for soups or stews, adding texture and flavor to meals.

As with any snack, it's important to practice mindful eating and enjoy pork rinds in moderation. While they can be a satisfying and nutrient-dense option, it's essential to incorporate a variety of foods in your carnivore diet to ensure a well-rounded and balanced approach.

Nourishing Bone Broth

Indulge in the comforting and nourishing experience of sipping on warm bone broth. This savory beverage has been cherished for centuries due to its numerous health benefits and rich nutrient profile. Bone broth is made by simmering bones and connective tissues of animals, such as beef, lamb, chicken, or fish, in water for an extended period, usually with the addition of aromatic vegetables and herbs.

One of the key benefits of bone broth is its abundant amino acid content. Amino acids are the building blocks of proteins and play vital roles in various physiological processes in the body. Bone broth is particularly rich in collagen, which is a protein that provides structure and support to the skin, bones, joints, and connective tissues. Consuming collagen-rich bone broth may promote joint health, improve skin elasticity, and support healthy hair and nails.

In addition to amino acids, bone broth is a good source of essential fatty acids, electrolytes, minerals, and trace elements. These nutrients contribute to overall health and wellness by supporting proper cellular function, electrolyte balance, and hydration. Bone broth is known for containing minerals like calcium, magnesium, phosphorus, and potassium, which are essential for bone health, muscle function, and maintaining a healthy nervous system.

Another noteworthy component of bone broth is gelatin, a substance that is formed during the cooking process when collagen breaks down. Gelatin is known for its soothing and gut-healing properties. It may support digestive health by promoting the integrity of the gut lining and reducing inflammation in the digestive tract. This makes bone broth a popular choice for individuals with gut-related issues or those looking to support their digestive system.

The slow and gentle simmering process used to make bone broth helps extract valuable nutrients from the bones and connective tissues. It also allows for the release of compounds such as glucosamine and chondroitin sulfate, which are known to support joint health and reduce inflammation. These compounds are often used as supplements for individuals with joint-related problems.

When selecting bone broth, it is important to choose high-quality options made from organic, grass-fed, or pasture-raised animal sources. This ensures that the broth is free from antibiotics, hormones, and other potentially harmful substances. Additionally, homemade bone broth prepared from scratch allows you to have control over the ingredients and cooking process, resulting in a truly nourishing and personalized beverage.

Bone broth can be enjoyed as a warm and comforting drink on its own or used as a base for soups, stews, and other recipes. It can be sipped throughout the day as a nourishing snack or incorporated into meals to enhance both the flavor and nutritional content.

Sardine Power

Embrace the nutritional prowess of canned sardines, a convenient and nutrient-dense snack that aligns with the principles of the carnivore diet. These small, oily fish are packed with a range of essential nutrients, making them an excellent choice to fuel your body and support optimal health.

One of the standout benefits of canned sardines is their high content of omega-3 fatty acids. These healthy fats, including EPA (eicosapentaenoic acid) and DHA (docosahexaenoic acid), play a crucial role in promoting heart health, supporting brain function, and reducing inflammation in the body. Omega-3 fatty acids have been associated with a lower risk of cardiovascular disease, improved cognitive function, and even mood regulation.

In addition to omega-3 fatty acids, sardines are a rich source of protein, which is essential for building and repairing tissues, supporting muscle growth, and maintaining overall bodily functions. Protein is made up of amino acids, which are the building blocks of life. Sardines provide a complete protein source, meaning they contain all the essential amino acids that your body needs but cannot produce on its own.

Canned sardines are also a great source of several vitamins and minerals. They are particularly rich in vitamin B12, which is important for red blood cell production, neurological function, and DNA synthesis. Sardines also contain significant amounts of vitamin D, which is crucial for bone health, immune function, and overall well-being. Other vitamins found in sardines include vitamin A, vitamin E, and various B vitamins. In terms of minerals, sardines are notably high in calcium, phosphorus, iron, magnesium, and selenium.

Furthermore, sardines are an excellent source of trace elements such as iodine and zinc. Iodine is essential for proper thyroid function and plays a vital role in regulating metabolism, growth, and development. Zinc is involved in numerous enzymatic reactions in the body, supporting immune function, wound healing, and cellular repair.

Choosing canned sardines as a snack ensures their long shelf life, easy portability, and versatility in incorporating them into your meals. Look for sardines that are canned in water or olive oil to avoid any unwanted additives or unhealthy fats. Opting for sustainably sourced sardines, such as those certified by reputable organizations like the Marine Stewardship Council (MSC), ensures that you are making an environmentally conscious choice.

To enjoy canned sardines as a snack, simply open the can and drain off any excess liquid or oil. They can be eaten directly from the can, or you can pair them with other carnivore-friendly ingredients like pork rinds or beef jerky for an added crunch and flavor.

Grilled Shrimp Delight

Treat yourself to the succulent flavors of grilled shrimp, a protein-rich snack that not only satisfies your taste buds but also offers a range of health benefits. Shrimp is a micronutrient-dense food that is low in calories and high in essential nutrients, making it a fantastic option for a quick and nutritious bite.

One of the key advantages of shrimp is its impressive protein content. Protein is an essential macronutrient that plays a crucial role in various bodily functions. It is responsible for building and repairing tissues, supporting muscle growth and maintenance, and aiding in the production of enzymes and hormones. Shrimp is a high-quality source of protein, providing all the essential amino acids your body needs for optimal health and well-being.

Despite being relatively low in calories, shrimp is rich in several important vitamins and minerals. It is particularly abundant in selenium, a trace mineral that acts as a powerful antioxidant, protecting cells from damage caused by free radicals. Selenium also plays a role in supporting thyroid function, immune health, and DNA synthesis. Additionally, shrimp contains notable amounts of vitamin B12, which is essential for nerve function, DNA synthesis, and the production of red blood cells.

Shrimp is also an excellent source of omega-3 fatty acids, including EPA (eicosapentaenoic acid) and DHA (docosahexaenoic acid). These omega-3 fatty acids are beneficial for heart health, as they help reduce inflammation, lower blood pressure, and improve overall cardiovascular function. They are also known to support brain health and cognitive function.

Furthermore, shrimp provides a range of other essential nutrients such as iodine, zinc, copper, and vitamin E. Iodine is necessary for proper thyroid function, while zinc and copper are involved in various enzymatic reactions in the body. Vitamin E is a potent antioxidant that helps protect cells from oxidative stress and supports immune function.

Grilling shrimp not only enhances its natural flavors but also helps retain its nutrient content. Grilling is a cooking method that requires minimal added fats, making it a healthier option compared to frying or deep-frying. To grill shrimp, simply marinate them in your choice of seasonings, skewer them, and cook them over medium heat until they are opaque and slightly charred. You can enjoy grilled shrimp as a standalone snack or alongside other carnivore-friendly ingredients for a satisfying meal.

When purchasing shrimp, opt for wild-caught or sustainably-farmed varieties whenever possible to ensure the best quality and minimize environmental impact. It's worth noting that individuals with shellfish allergies should avoid shrimp or any other shellfish products.

Bone Marrow Treat

Treat yourself to the indulgent and nutritious delight of bone marrow. Often considered a delicacy, bone marrow is not only rich in flavor but also packed with a variety of beneficial nutrients, making it a standout choice for those following the carnivore diet.

Bone marrow is the soft, fatty substance found within the hollow center of bones. It is a concentrated source of healthy fats, particularly monounsaturated fats and omega-3 fatty acids. These fats play a vital role in supporting heart health, reducing inflammation, and promoting proper brain function. Including bone marrow in your diet can help provide the essential fatty acids needed for optimal well-being.

In addition to healthy fats, bone marrow is a noteworthy source of several key vitamins and minerals. It is particularly rich in vitamins A and K. Vitamin A is essential for maintaining healthy vision, promoting immune function, and supporting skin health. Vitamin K is crucial for blood clotting, bone health, and the proper functioning of various enzymes in the body.

Bone marrow is also a good source of iron, zinc, and phosphorus. Iron is essential for oxygen transport and energy production, while zinc plays a vital role in immune function, cell growth, and wound healing. Phosphorus is necessary for healthy bones and teeth, energy metabolism, and the formation of DNA.

To enjoy bone marrow, it is typically roasted or boiled, which helps soften the marrow and enhance its flavors. The rich, creamy texture and buttery taste make it a delightful addition to various dishes. You can spread it on beef burgers, use it as a flavorful ingredient in sauces and soups, or simply enjoy it on its own.

When sourcing bone marrow, it is important to choose high-quality, grass-fed or pasture-raised sources whenever possible. This ensures that the animals have been raised in a natural and healthy environment, promoting the nutritional quality of the marrow.

Pemmican Energy

Experience the energy-boosting power of pemmican, a traditional Native American food that has been enjoyed for centuries. Pemmican is a nutrient-dense snack that combines dried meat with rendered fat, creating a portable and high-energy food source that provides sustenance and satiety.

The process of making pemmican involves drying lean meat, such as beef, bison, or venison, to remove the moisture content. This preservation technique not only extends the shelf life of the meat but also concentrates its nutrients. The dried meat is then pounded or shredded into fine pieces.

To enhance the nutritional profile and improve the taste, rendered fat is added to the dried meat. The fat can come from various sources, including beef tallow, suet, or even bone marrow. The fat acts as a binder, holding the meat together and providing a rich source of energy.

Pemmican is prized for its high energy density, making it an excellent choice for individuals needing a quick and convenient source of nourishment. The combination of protein from the dried meat and the healthy fats from the rendered fat provides a well-rounded macronutrient composition that can sustain physical activity and support overall well-being.

The nutritional benefits of pemmican extend beyond its macronutrient content. It is a rich source of essential vitamins and minerals, including iron, zinc, and B-vitamins. Iron is crucial for oxygen transport and energy production, while zinc plays a vital role in immune function, metabolism, and wound healing. B-vitamins are involved in various bodily processes, including energy production and brain function.

Moreover, pemmican's high-fat content provides a concentrated source of calories, which can be particularly beneficial for those on low-carbohydrate or ketogenic diets. The healthy fats in pemmican, such as monounsaturated and saturated fats, are a valuable source of energy and help promote satiety.

The portability of pemmican makes it an ideal snack for outdoor activities, long hikes, or situations where access to fresh food is limited. Its long shelf life and resistance to spoilage make it a reliable option for emergency food supplies or survival situations.

When choosing pemmican, it is essential to opt for high-quality sources that use organic, grass-fed, or pasture-raised meats. This ensures that the meat used is of superior quality, free from antibiotics or hormones, and higher in beneficial nutrients. Additionally, it's important to be mindful of the fat source, opting for healthy fats that are minimally processed.

Steak Tartare Adventure

Embark on a culinary journey by trying the exquisite delicacy known as steak tartare. This extraordinary dish is a testament to the art of raw food preparation and highlights the natural goodness of high-quality beef in a way that is both captivating and delicious.

Steak tartare is traditionally made using finely chopped or minced raw beef, sourced from the finest cuts of meat.

The meat is carefully selected for its freshness, tenderness, and flavor. It is important to choose meat from trusted sources, ensuring that it is of the highest quality and handled with proper food safety practices.

The raw beef is then seasoned with an array of spices, herbs, and condiments, which may vary depending on personal preference and regional culinary traditions. Common ingredients used to enhance the flavor profile of steak tartare include finely chopped onions, capers, Dijon mustard, Worcestershire sauce, fresh herbs like parsley or chives, and a hint of acidity from lemon juice or vinegar. These seasonings work harmoniously to elevate the taste and create a unique culinary experience.

One of the key elements that distinguishes steak tartare is its texture. The finely chopped beef provides a tender yet substantial mouthfeel, allowing you to savor the natural juiciness and richness of the meat. The delicate balance of flavors, combined with the satisfying texture, makes every bite a sensory delight.

When consuming raw meat, it is crucial to prioritize food safety and hygiene. The meat used for steak tartare should come from trusted sources and be handled with the utmost care to minimize the risk of foodborne illnesses. Proper refrigeration, storage, and handling practices should be followed to maintain the freshness and safety of the ingredients.

Steak tartare is not only a culinary adventure but also a nutritional powerhouse. High-quality beef is an excellent source of protein, essential amino acids, vitamins, minerals, and trace elements. It is particularly rich in nutrients like iron, zinc, and B-vitamins, which are vital for various bodily functions, including energy production, immune support, and tissue repair.

It's important to note that not everyone may be suited for consuming raw meat, and individuals with compromised immune systems or certain health conditions should exercise caution. Pregnant women, young children, and the elderly should consult with a healthcare professional before indulging in raw meat dishes.

For those venturing into the world of steak tartare, it is recommended to try it at reputable establishments known for their expertise in preparing raw meat dishes. Alternatively, with proper knowledge and skills in handling raw meat, it can be prepared at home using the freshest and highest-quality ingredients.

Delectable Bacon

Treat yourself to the irresistible allure of dehydrated bacon, a snack that combines convenience with the unmistakable flavors of smoky and crispy goodness. Dehydrated bacon offers a unique twist on this beloved meat, providing a concentrated burst of flavor that satisfies cravings and delivers a satisfying crunch.

To create dehydrated bacon, high-quality bacon strips are carefully prepared and subjected to a controlled dehydration process. This process involves removing the moisture from the bacon while preserving its flavor, aroma, and texture. The result is a lightweight and shelf-stable snack that retains the essence of bacon in a concentrated form.

Dehydrated bacon not only offers a convenient and portable snack option but also intensifies the flavors that bacon enthusiasts adore. The dehydration process concentrates the smoky, savory, and slightly sweet taste of bacon, enhancing its natural richness. Each bite provides a satisfying crunch that adds a pleasant texture to the snacking experience.

As with any bacon product, it is crucial to choose high-quality bacon from reputable sources. Opting for bacon sourced from humanely raised pigs, preferably free from antibiotics and added hormones, ensures not only a superior flavor but also aligns with ethical and sustainable food choices.

As part of a carnivore or keto lifestyle, dehydrated bacon can provide a great source of satiating fats and proteins. When enjoying dehydrated bacon, consider pairing it with other carnivore-friendly snacks or incorporating it into recipes to add a flavorful twist. It can be used as a topping for salads, a crunchy addition to soups or stews, or a protein-packed ingredient in homemade trail mix. The versatility of dehydrated bacon allows you to explore various creative ways to incorporate it into your culinary repertoire.

It's worth noting that while dehydrated bacon offers convenience and intense flavor, it does not provide the same texture as traditional cooked bacon. The absence of fat rendering during dehydration results in a crisper and drier texture. Embracing this unique texture can enhance the snacking experience and open up new avenues for culinary experimentation.

Cheese Pleasures

Indulge in the vast array of cheese options available to elevate your carnivore diet snacking experience. Cheese, a versatile and flavorful dairy product, not only satisfies your taste buds but also offers a host of nutritional benefits. With its rich profile of protein, healthy fats, vitamins, minerals, and trace elements, cheese serves as a delightful and satiating addition to your carnivore repertoire.

One of the primary attractions of cheese is its creamy and savory nature, which lends itself well to snacking. The diverse range of flavors and textures found in different cheese varieties allows you to explore and discover your personal preferences. From mild and soft cheeses like brie and mozzarella to sharp and aged ones like cheddar and Parmesan, there is a cheese to suit every palate.

Cheese is a notable source of protein, providing essential amino acids necessary for building and repairing tissues in the body. It offers a complete protein profile, making it particularly beneficial for those following a carnivore diet. Protein plays a crucial role in muscle development, satiety, and overall bodily functions, making cheese an excellent snack choice to support your dietary goals.

Furthermore, cheese is rich in healthy fats, including saturated fats and monounsaturated fats. These fats contribute to the creamy texture and rich flavor of cheese while providing a source of energy. Saturated fats, in particular, are essential for hormone production, brain function, and cell membrane integrity. Contrary to previous misconceptions, research suggests that natural saturated fats from sources like cheese can be part of a healthy diet.

In addition to protein and healthy fats, cheese contains a variety of essential vitamins and minerals. These include calcium, which is crucial for bone health and muscle function, as well as phosphorus, which supports proper cell function and energy metabolism. Cheese also provides vitamins such as vitamin A, important for vision and immune function, and vitamin B12, essential for nerve function and red blood cell production.

When incorporating cheese into your carnivore snacking routine, it's important to consider the quality and sourcing of the cheese. Opt for cheeses made from high-quality milk, preferably sourced from grass-fed or pasture-raised animals. These cheeses tend to have a more favorable nutritional profile, with higher levels of omega-3 fatty acids and beneficial conjugated linoleic acid (CLA).

Keep in mind that cheese can be very calorie-dense, so it's important to be mindful of portion sizes in order to maintain a calorie balance. Additionally, some individuals may have sensitivities or intolerances to certain types of cheese or dairy products. If you experience any adverse effects, it's best to consult with a healthcare professional.

Whether enjoyed on its own, paired with other carnivore-friendly snacks, or incorporated into recipes, cheese provides a satisfying, nutritious, and flavorful snacking experience. From cheese boards showcasing a variety of flavors to simple cheese cubes for a quick bite, there are endless possibilities to explore.

Protein-packed Eggs

Hard-boiled eggs, a timeless classic, are an exceptional snack choice for carnivores seeking a convenient and nutrient-dense option. Eggs are renowned for their high protein content, providing all the essential amino acids necessary for various physiological functions in the body. This protein powerhouse supports muscle growth, repair, and maintenance, making it an excellent choice for individuals following a carnivore diet.

In addition to protein, eggs boast an impressive nutrient profile. They are a rich source of essential vitamins, including vitamin A, vitamin D, vitamin E, vitamin K, and various B vitamins, such as vitamin B12, riboflavin, and folate. These vitamins play critical roles in energy metabolism, cellular function, neurological health, and the production of red blood cells. Incorporating hard-boiled eggs into your snacking routine can contribute to meeting your daily vitamin requirements.

Minerals and trace elements are also abundantly found in eggs. They contain essential minerals like iron, zinc, phosphorus, and selenium, which are necessary for various physiological processes. Iron is vital for oxygen transport and plays a crucial role in preventing iron-deficiency anemia. Zinc is involved in immune function, wound healing, and DNA synthesis, while phosphorus is essential for bone health and energy production. Selenium acts as an antioxidant, protecting cells from oxidative damage and supporting thyroid function.

Moreover, eggs are a natural source of antioxidants, such as lutein and zeaxanthin, which are beneficial for eye health and may reduce the risk of age-related macular degeneration. These antioxidants help neutralize harmful free radicals, reducing oxidative stress and promote overall well-being.

When selecting eggs, consider choosing pasture-raised or organic options whenever possible. These eggs are typically sourced from hens that have access to a natural diet and are not treated with hormones or antibiotics. They tend to contain higher levels of beneficial nutrients like omega-3 fatty acids, which support heart health and brain function.

Hard-boiled eggs are an incredibly versatile snack that can be enjoyed on their own or used as a base for various creative recipes. You can sprinkle them with a pinch of sea salt or pepper for added flavor, or even experiment with different seasonings and herbs. If desired, you can also pair them with other carnivore-approved snacks, like bacon, cheese, or jerky for a well-rounded snacking experience.

Liver Crisps

For a unique and nutrient-packed snack, consider trying liver crisps. Made by thinly slicing and dehydrating liver, this snack offers a delightful crunch and an impressive array of vitamins and minerals essential for optimal health.

Liver is often hailed as a nutritional powerhouse due to its concentrated nutrient content. It is an abundant source of vitamin A, a fat-soluble vitamin that plays a vital role in maintaining healthy vision, supporting immune function, and promoting cellular growth and differentiation. Vitamin A is also essential for the health of epithelial tissues, such as the skin and mucous membranes, and contributes to overall skin integrity.

Another notable nutrient found in liver is vitamin B12, which is crucial for red blood cell production, neurological function, and DNA synthesis. This vitamin is primarily found in animal-based foods, making liver an excellent choice for individuals following the carnivore diet. Adequate intake of vitamin B12 is essential for preventing deficiencies and supporting optimal cognitive function.

Liver is also rich in iron, a mineral that is integral to the formation of hemoglobin, the protein responsible for carrying oxygen throughout the body. Iron is vital for preventing iron-deficiency anemia and supporting energy metabolism. Additionally, liver contains copper, a trace mineral involved in the production and maintenance of connective tissue, iron absorption, and antioxidant defence.

Incorporating liver crisps into your snacking routine can provide a convenient and enjoyable way to boost your intake of these essential nutrients. The dehydration process preserves the nutritional integrity of liver while creating a satisfyingly crisp texture. Liver crisps can be enjoyed on their own or paired with other carnivore-friendly snacks, such as jerky or cheese, for a more diverse flavor experience.

Side Dishes

Cheesy Goodness

Enhance your meals with the addition of cheese as a flavorful and creamy side dish. Choose from a variety of cheese options to complement your carnivore diet. Cheese, with its rich and creamy texture, is a versatile and delicious addition to the carnivore diet. It not only provides flavor and satisfaction to meals but also offers several nutritional benefits. Here are some ways you can incorporate cheese as a side dish:

• **Cheese Platter:** Create a mouthwatering cheese platter with an assortment of your favorite cheeses. Choose from options like cheddar, Gouda, Swiss, mozzarella, or blue cheese. Pair them with cured meats, such as prosciutto or salami, for a delightful combination of flavors and textures.

• **Cheese Sauce:** Make a velvety cheese sauce to drizzle over your meat or vegetables. Melt cheese with heavy cream or butter for a creamy and indulgent sauce. You can customize the flavor by adding spices or herbs like garlic, paprika, or rosemary.

• **Cheese Crisps:** Create crispy and savory cheese crisps by baking or frying thin slices of cheese. Simply place small mounds of grated or sliced cheese on a baking sheet and bake until golden and crisp. These cheese crisps can be enjoyed on their own or used as a crunchy topping for salads or soups.

• **Cheese Stuffed Meat:** Elevate your carnivore meals by stuffing meat with cheese. For example, you can stuff chicken breast with mozzarella or wrap a steak around a filling of blue cheese. As the meat cooks, the cheese melts, creating a delicious and gooey center.

• **Cheese Melt:** Top your grilled meat or burgers with a slice of cheese to add extra flavor and creaminess. Let the cheese melt over the hot meat, creating a luscious coating.

Experiment with different cheese varieties to find your favorite combination.

• **Cheese Roll-Ups:** Create roll-ups using cheese as a base. Wrap slices of meat, such as ham or roast beef, around a strip of cheese to create a satisfying and protein-rich snack or appetizer.

Cheese is not only a source of protein but also provides essential nutrients such as calcium, phosphorus, and vitamins, like vitamin B12 and vitamin K2. It adds a delightful burst of flavor to meals and can be enjoyed in various forms, making it a versatile choice for the carnivore diet.

Creamy Indulgence

Elevate the flavor and texture of your carnivore meals by incorporating heavy cream as a side dish. This luscious and decadent ingredient not only enhances the taste of your dishes but also provides a valuable source of healthy fats.

Heavy cream, also known as heavy whipping cream, is derived from the high-fat layer of cow's milk. It is rich in beneficial fats, particularly saturated fats and monounsaturated fats, which are important for various functions in the body. These fats provide a concentrated source of energy, aid in the absorption of fat-soluble vitamins, support hormone production, and contribute to the feeling of satiety after a meal.

In addition to its fat content, heavy cream adds a creamy and velvety texture to dishes, making them more satisfying and enjoyable. Whether you drizzle it over a sizzling steak, blend it into scrambled eggs, or whisk it into a sauce, heavy cream lends a luxurious mouthfeel and enhances the overall dining experience.

Furthermore, heavy cream is a versatile ingredient that can be used in both sweet and savory preparations. It can be whipped into fluffy peaks to top desserts or used as a base for homemade ice creams and custards. On the savory side, it can be incorporated into creamy soups, sauces, or mashed cauliflower to add depth and richness to the flavors.

When selecting heavy cream, it is ideal to opt for organic or grass-fed varieties whenever possible. These options are sourced from cows that have been raised in more natural and sustainable environments, resulting in a higher nutrient content and a better fatty acid profile.

Eggcellent Choice

When it comes to enhancing the protein content and adding a touch of richness to your carnivore meals, eggs are an excellent choice. Not only are they incredibly versatile, but they also offer a wide array of essential nutrients that can support your overall health and well-being.

Eggs are known for being a complete protein source, meaning they contain all the essential amino acids your body needs for various physiological functions, including muscle repair and growth. Additionally, eggs are packed with vitamins and minerals, such as vitamin A, vitamin D, vitamin E, vitamin B12, riboflavin, folate, iron, and selenium, to name just a few. These nutrients play crucial roles in energy production, immune function, and maintaining healthy bones, among other benefits.

When considering eggs as a side dish, you have numerous preparation options to suit your preferences. You can enjoy them hard-boiled, soft-boiled, poached, scrambled, or fried. Each method offers a unique texture and flavor profile that can add variety to your carnivore meals. Furthermore, incorporating egg yolks specifically can provide an extra dose of nutrients and healthy fats.

Egg yolks are a concentrated source of essential vitamins, such as vitamin A, vitamin D, vitamin E, and vitamin K2, which are important for vision, bone health, immune function, and cardiovascular health. They also contain choline, a nutrient that supports brain health and development.

One delicious way to incorporate eggs or egg yolks as a side dish is by creating a homemade hollandaise sauce. This rich and creamy sauce, made with egg yolks, butter, and lemon juice, can be drizzled over steak, fish, or roasted vegetables, adding a luxurious touch and a burst of flavor.

Bacon Bliss

Indulge in the mouthwatering delight of crispy bacon as a side dish to elevate the flavor and texture of your carnivore meals. Bacon, derived from cured and smoked pork belly, adds a distinct savory and smoky element that can enhance the overall taste experience of your dishes.

When it comes to bacon, its appeal goes beyond just its delicious flavor. It also contributes to the enjoyment and satisfaction of your meals. The crispiness of properly cooked bacon provides a satisfying crunch that adds texture to your carnivore dishes.

In addition to its irresistible taste and texture, bacon offers a source of high-quality protein and essential fats. Protein is crucial for building and repairing tissues, supporting muscle growth, and maintaining overall health. It also helps keep you feeling satiated and satisfied after meals. The fat content in bacon consists of a combination of monounsaturated and saturated fats, which are necessary for hormone production, insulation of organs, and absorption of fat-soluble vitamins.

Bacon is also a source of important nutrients, including vitamins and minerals. It contains notable amounts of vitamins B1, B2, B3, B5, B6, and B12, as well as minerals like iron, zinc, magnesium, and selenium. These nutrients play essential roles in energy metabolism, immune function, and overall well-being.

When incorporating bacon as a side dish, you have the flexibility to pair it with various carnivore-friendly main courses. It can be served alongside grilled steak, roasted chicken, or even as a complement to eggs for a hearty breakfast. Crumbled bacon can also be used to top salads, soups, or vegetables, providing a burst of flavor and a satisfying crunch.

Seafood Delights

Embark on a culinary journey and embrace the diverse flavors and textures that seafood offers by including options like shrimp, smoked salmon, or other delectable seafood as side dishes in your carnivore meals. These oceanic treasures not only provide a delightful taste experience but also contribute an array of essential nutrients to support your overall health and well-being.

Shrimp, a popular crustacean, is a fantastic choice to add to your carnivore diet. It is low in calories and carbohydrates, making it a great option for those following a low-carb lifestyle. Shrimp is also an excellent source of high-quality protein, which is essential for tissue repair, muscle maintenance, and numerous enzymatic functions in the body. Additionally, shrimp contains an abundance of essential minerals, including selenium, copper, zinc, and magnesium, which are vital for various physiological processes, such as immune function, metabolism, and bone health.

Another seafood option to savor is smoked salmon. This delicacy undergoes a smoking process that imparts a rich, savory flavor and tender texture to the fish. Smoked salmon is not only a culinary delight, but also a valuable source of heart-healthy omega-3 fatty acids. These omega-3 fats, particularly EPA and DHA, play a crucial role in reducing inflammation, supporting brain function, and promoting cardiovascular health. Smoked salmon is also rich in protein, B vitamins, vitamin D, and minerals like selenium and phosphorus.

By incorporating a variety of seafood options into your carnivore meals, you can further diversify your nutrient intake. Different types of fish and shellfish offer a wide range of nutrients, including vitamins, minerals, and trace elements. For example, shellfish such as mussels, oysters, and crabs are excellent sources of iron, zinc, copper, and vitamin B12. These nutrients are essential for red blood cell production, immune function, and nerve health.

To enjoy these seafood delights as side dishes, you can pair them with grilled meat, steak, or other carnivore main courses. Shrimp can be sautéed with herbs and spices or grilled to perfection. Smoked salmon can be enjoyed as is or incorporated into salads or omelets for a burst of flavor. Experimenting with different seafood options allows you to explore new tastes and textures while reaping their exceptional nutritional benefits.

When selecting seafood, opt for wild-caught or sustainably farmed options to ensure their quality, minimize environmental impact, and support sustainable fishing practices. Freshness is also key, as it guarantees optimal flavor and nutrient content.

Bone Marrow Elixir

Indulge in the velvety richness and nutrient-packed elixir that is bone marrow. This culinary delight not only adds a burst of flavor to your carnivore meals but also offers a treasure trove of essential nutrients that support optimal health and well-being.

Bone marrow is the soft, fatty tissue found within the bones of animals, and it is known for its exquisite taste and unique texture. When cooked, bone marrow transforms into a luscious, buttery substance that can be spread on meat, used as a flavorful sauce, or enjoyed on its own. It is a versatile addition to your carnivore diet, enhancing the taste and satiety of your meals.

From a nutritional standpoint, bone marrow is a powerhouse. It is rich in healthy fats, including monounsaturated fats and omega-3 fatty acids, which are beneficial for heart health, brain function, and inflammation regulation. These fats are essential for the absorption of fat-soluble vitamins, such as vitamins A, D, E, and K, which are abundant in bone marrow.

Speaking of vitamins, bone marrow is a concentrated source of various essential vitamins and minerals. It is particularly high in vitamin A, which is vital for vision, immune function, and cellular growth. Bone marrow also provides significant amounts of vitamin K, which plays a crucial role in blood clotting and bone health. Additionally, it contains minerals like calcium, phosphorus, magnesium, and zinc, all of which are essential for proper bone formation, muscle function, and immune support.

Incorporating bone marrow as a side dish in your carnivore meals not only elevates the flavor profile but also contributes to a well-rounded nutrient intake. To enjoy this delicacy, you can roast bone marrow bones in the oven until the marrow becomes soft and scoopable. Then, spread it on cooked meat or use it as a dip for a savory indulgence. You can also use bone marrow as a base for sauces or incorporate it into soups and stews to add depth and richness to your dishes.

When selecting bone marrow, opt for high-quality sources such as grass-fed or pasture-raised animals. This ensures that the marrow comes from animals raised in natural and humane conditions, yielding superior taste and nutrient composition.

Savoring the bone marrow elixir as a side dish adds a touch of luxury and nourishment to your carnivore meals. With its delectable taste and abundant nutrients, bone marrow is a culinary gem that offers a host of health benefits.

Organ Meat Powerhouse

Elevate your carnivore meals with the nutritional powerhouses that are organ meats. While often overlooked, organ meats such as beef or chicken liver, heart, and other organs offer a wealth of essential nutrients that can significantly enhance your overall health and well-being, and promote longevity.

Organ meats are highly concentrated sources of vitamins, minerals, and bioactive compounds. They are particularly rich in B vitamins, including vitamin B12, which is essential for nerve function, DNA synthesis, and red blood cell production. Organ meats also provide ample amounts of vitamin A, which promotes healthy vision, immune function, and skin health. Moreover, they contain minerals like iron, zinc, copper, and selenium, which are critical for energy production, immune support, and antioxidant defence.

Incorporating organ meats into your carnivore diet introduces a wide array of beneficial compounds that support optimal health. For instance, liver is an excellent source of bioavailable iron, making it especially beneficial for individuals at risk of iron deficiency or anemia. It also contains unique compounds like choline, which plays a crucial role in brain development, liver function, and metabolism.

Heart, another nutrient-dense organ meat, is abundant in coenzyme Q10 (CoQ10), a potent antioxidant that supports cardiovascular health and energy production at the cellular level. It also contains essential amino acid-like compounds, like taurine and carnitine, which contribute to heart health and promote efficient energy metabolism.

When preparing organ meats as side dishes, it's important to choose high-quality, pasture-raised or grass-fed sources to ensure the highest nutrient content and minimize exposure to potential toxins or antibiotics. While organ meats have distinct flavors, they can be prepared in various ways to suit your taste preferences. They can be pan-fried, grilled, roasted, or added to stews and casseroles, offering a delicious and nutrient-packed addition to your carnivore meals.

If you're new to incorporating organ meats into your diet, start with smaller portions and gradually increase your intake as you become more accustomed to their flavors. Experiment with different cooking techniques and seasonings to find the combinations that best suit your palate.

Shellfish Sensations

Elevate your carnivore meals with the exquisite flavors and exceptional nutrient profiles of shellfish. Scallops, mussels, oysters, crabs, and lobsters not only add a touch of elegance to your plate, but also offer a treasure trove of essential minerals and omega-3 fatty acids that contribute to your overall health.

Shellfish are renowned for their micronutrient content, providing significant amounts of minerals, such as zinc, copper, selenium, and iron. Zinc plays a vital role in immune function, wound healing, and protein synthesis, while copper is involved in energy production, antioxidant defence, and connective tissue formation. Selenium acts as a powerful antioxidant, supporting thyroid function and immune system health. Iron is crucial for oxygen transport and energy metabolism.

Moreover, shellfish are excellent sources of omega-3 fatty acids, particularly in the form of eicosapentaenoic acid (EPA) and docosahexaenoic acid (DHA). These essential fatty acids are renowned for their anti-inflammatory properties and their roles in supporting heart health, joint health, brain function, and optimal immune response. Including shellfish in your carnivore diet helps ensure an adequate intake of these beneficial fats.

Each type of shellfish offers its own unique nutritional profile. Scallops, for example, are an exceptional source of protein, magnesium, and potassium, which support muscle function and cardiovascular health. Mussels are rich in vitamin B12, selenium, and manganese, all of which contribute to energy production, brain health, and antioxidant defence. Oysters are prized for their high zinc content, which supports immune function, hormonal balance, sexual performance, and reproductive health. Crabs provide an abundance of vitamin B12, phosphorus, and selenium, vital for energy metabolism, bone health, and antioxidant activity. Lobsters boast an impressive array of nutrients, including vitamin B12, copper, and zinc, supporting nerve function, red blood cell production, and immune health.

When incorporating shellfish as side dishes, opt for fresh, high-quality sources to ensure optimal flavor and nutrient content. Enjoy them steamed, grilled, roasted, or in delicious seafood stews and soups. Be mindful of any potential allergies or sensitivities to shellfish, and if you're unsure, consult with a healthcare professional.

Summary

By exploring these diverse meal ideas, snacks, and side dishes, you can experience the full range of flavors, textures, and nutritional benefits that the carnivore diet has to offer. Remember to prioritize high-quality ingredients and enjoy the bountiful benefits of a carnivorous or animal-based way of eating.

7-Day Carnivore Diet Meal Plan

Getting started with the carnivore diet is easy if you have a pre-designed diet plan available to you. You may use the following 7-day carnivore diet meal plan as your starting guide:

Day 1

- Breakfast: Ribeye steak
- Lunch: Ground beef patties
- Dinner: Salmon fillet

Day 2

- Breakfast: Bacon and eggs (a breakfast classic)
- Lunch: Chicken thighs
- Dinner: Pork chops

Day 3

- Breakfast: Sausage links
- Lunch: Tuna steak
- Dinner: Lamb chops

Day 4

- Breakfast: Steak and eggs (great for body recomposition)
- Lunch: Turkey breast
- Dinner: Bison burgers

Day 5

- Breakfast: Ham steak
- Lunch: Venison steak
- Dinner: Chicken wings

Day 6

- Breakfast: Ground lamb omelet
- Lunch: Beef liver
- Dinner: Shrimp skewers

Day 7

- Breakfast: Pork belly strips
- Lunch: Duck breast
- Dinner: Prime rib roast

Remember to season your meats with salt, pepper, and other approved spices for added flavor. It's important to prioritize high-quality, grass-fed, or pasture-raised meats whenever possible.

This 7-day carnivore diet meal plan provides a variety of meat options to keep your meals interesting and enjoyable while staying compliant with the principles of the carnivore diet. Feel free to customize it based on your personal preferences and dietary needs.

Eating Out and Traveling on the Carnivore Diet

Following the carnivore diet can present certain challenges when it comes to eating out and travelling. However, with a little bit of planning and knowledge, it is possible to maintain the carnivore lifestyle successfully while enjoying delicious meals at restaurants and staying on track during your travels.

In this subchapter, we will explore some powerful strategies and tips for navigating restaurants, finding suitable options, and even cooking on the go when following the carnivore diet, allowing you to adhere to it successfully without sacrificing your dietary needs, priorities, and health goals.

Eating Out on the Carnivore Diet

When dining out, it is important to communicate your dietary preferences clearly to the waitstaff or server. Many restaurants are accommodating and can offer a range of carnivore-friendly options. One useful approach is to look for an "a la carte" option on the menu, where you can order individual meat items without any accompanying sides or carbohydrates. This allows you to customize your meal to fit your unique dietary needs.

Burger chains can also be a reliable choice, as they typically offer the option to order multiple burger patties.

You can enhance the flavor by adding cheese or bacon for added fat and enjoyment. Additionally, some fast-food restaurants allow you to order multiple sides of meat, making it easier to get an adequate protein intake.

When dining at Mexican or Tex-Mex restaurants, opt for fajitas or grilled meats without any tortillas or sides. Chipotle, a popular fast-casual chain in the United States, offers the flexibility to order a bowl with multiple meat options, providing a rich and satisfying carnivore-compliant meal.

Staying on Track While Traveling

Traveling while following the carnivore diet can present additional challenges, but with some preparation, you can maintain compliance successfully. For example, when booking accommodations, consider choosing a hotel or rental with a kitchenette or access to a kitchen. This allows you to cook your own meals and have more control over the ingredients and cooking methods. Sous vide devices are portable and convenient for cooking delicious, slow-roasted meats, like prime rib, without the need for an oven or causing smoke.

If cooking isn't an option, research carnivore-friendly restaurants or grocery stores at your destination. In larger cities, you are more likely to find restaurants that cater to various dietary preferences, including carnivore options. Utilize online resources and apps that provide reviews and recommendations to find suitable eateries.

During air travel, it can be challenging to find carnivore-friendly options at airports or on flights. Packing your own food is a great solution to this. Bring pre-cooked meats, like jerky or pemmican, hard-boiled eggs, and canned fish, like sardines or tuna. These portable options provide nutrient-dense and satiating choices for your carnivore journey.

When dining out or travelling internationally, it is crucial to be mindful of the quality of the meat you consume. Aim for grass-fed or pasture-raised meats whenever possible, as they are more nutrient-dense and offer a better balance of fatty acids (omega-3s vs. omega-6s). Local markets or butcher shops can be excellent resources for obtaining high-quality meats.

Examples of What To Order At Restaurants

When dining out, there are several delicious carnivore options to choose from. Here are some examples of carnivore-friendly dishes you can order at different types of restaurants:

1. Steak: A classic choice for carnivores, steak is a staple at many restaurants. Opt for fatty cuts like ribeye, New York strip, or porterhouse. Pair it with a side of grass-fed butter for added flavor and richness.

2. **Burger Patties:** Many burger chains offer the flexibility to order multiple burger patties without the bun or any condiments. Customize your burger by adding cheese, bacon, or other preferred toppings to enhance the taste and satisfy your carnivorous cravings.

3. **Ribs:** Indulge in tender, slow-cooked ribs without worrying about sugary sauces or rubs. Look for restaurants that specialize in barbecue or smokehouses, as they often offer succulent pork or beef ribs seasoned with salt and pepper or dry rubs.

4. **Rotisserie Chicken:** Rotisserie chicken is a flavorful and convenient choice when dining out. Seek out establishments that offer rotisserie chicken as part of their menu. Opt for plain, unseasoned versions to avoid any unwanted ingredients.

5. **Seafood:** Seafood options can be an excellent choice for carnivores. Look for dishes like grilled salmon, seared tuna, or broiled shrimp. Avoid breaded or fried seafood and opt for simple preparations that highlight the natural flavors of these amazingly nutritious foods.

6. **Barbecue:** Barbecue joints are a carnivore dieter's paradise, offering a wide variety of smoked meats. Choose options like brisket, pulled pork, sausage, pulled chicken, or ribs. Be cautious of any barbecue sauces, as they often contain added sugars. Consider enjoying the meats on their own or with a side of vinegar-based sauce.

7. **Chicken Wings:** Ordering chicken wings can be a great way to enjoy a carnivore-friendly meal. Choose

wings without any breading or sugary sauces. Opt for traditional flavors, like buffalo or plain wings, and pair them with a side of ranch or blue cheese dressing.

8. Mexican Cuisine: Mexican restaurants can provide ample choices for carnivores. Look for dishes like carne asada (grilled steak), carnitas (slow-cooked pork), or barbacoa (slow-cooked beef). Skip the tortillas, rice, and beans altogether, and ask for extra servings of meat of your choice.

9. Mediterranean Cuisine: Mediterranean restaurants offer various grilled meat options that are suitable for those following the carnivore diet. Enjoy dishes like beef or chicken kabobs seasoned with herbs and spices. Pair them with a side of grilled cheese or smoked sausage.

Tip: It's always helpful to communicate your dietary preferences/needs to the restaurant staff when placing your order. They are often accommodating and willing to tailor dishes to suit your specific requirements.

Additionally, be mindful of any sauces, dressings, or marinades that may contain added sugars or undesirable ingredients.

By exploring different types of restaurants and choosing suitable items from their menus, you can continue to enjoy dining out while staying compliant with the carnivore diet's principles.

Key Points

• Eating out and travelling on the carnivore diet may require some additional planning and research, but it is entirely feasible to maintain compliance.

• Clear communication with restaurant staff, looking for customizable options, and opting for a la carte selections are effective strategies when dining out.

• During travel, having access to a kitchen or packing nutrient-dense, portable meat options can ensure you stay on track.

• Embracing the carnivore lifestyle doesn't mean compromising on taste or enjoyment while exploring new culinary experiences or visiting unfamiliar places. By being prepared, proactive, and open to adaptation, you can make the most of eating out and travelling on the carnivore diet.

5 Mistakes to Avoid When First Starting The Carnivore Diet

Navigating the carnivore diet with confidence requires a keen awareness of potential stumbling blocks that may impede your progress. To ensure a successful start to your carnivore journey, it is crucial to be mindful of the following mistakes that can hinder your results:

1. Sneaking in small amounts of fruits and vegetables: Some people don't fully understand the concept of "carnivore" and think that as long as their main source of nutrition comes from meat, everything is fine. That's not how this diet works. It's called the "carnivore diet" for a reason, so stick with animal products only.

2. Only buying lean cuts: Meat is available in lean and fatty cuts. You don't have to eat pork belly every day (pork belly is one of the fattiest cuts of meat), but please, don't be afraid of animal fat. Animal fat is what will provide your body with the fuel and nutrients it needs to thrive and heal.

3. Drinking too little water: Inadequate hydration can be a common pitfall when starting any dietary regimen, including the carnivore diet. Since the carnivore diet involves consuming a smaller volume of food and excludes water-rich fruits and vegetables, it is important to consciously increase your water intake. Additionally, supplementing with electrolytes, such as potassium, sodium, magnesium, calcium, and chloride can help, as plain water does not contain these vital electrolytes necessary for intracellular hydration. Maintaining proper hydration levels with electrolyte-rich fluids, including bone broth and electrolyte-infused water, promotes optimal metabolic function, aids digestion, and supports mood and energy levels.

4. Not eating enough: The carnivore diet is not about eating a little bit of meat here and there. You need to eat a decent amount of it, ideally, until you're full. Even if you are only interested in weight loss, your body still needs plenty of energy to keep working and keep your metabolic engines running.

5. Not adding salt: Electrolytes are vital for the salinity of your blood. When you eat just meat and no carbs or fiber, you may experience a drop in your body's electrolyte levels. For that reason, you shouldn't be afraid to salt your meals liberally and even salt your water if you have to. Staying well-hydrated is very important for mood, energy, digestive health, and more.

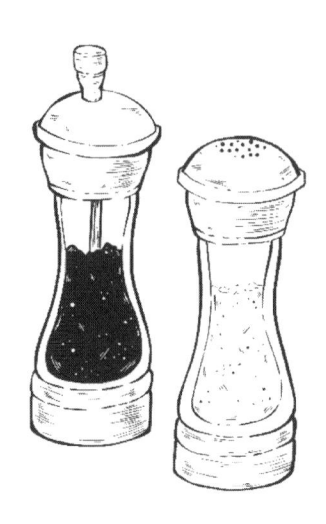

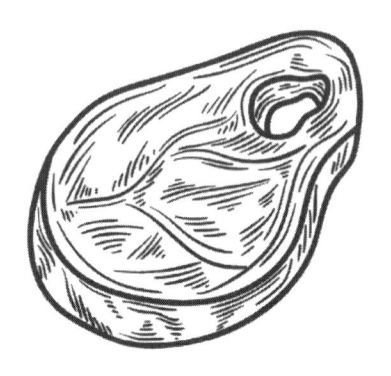

CHAPTER 2: RED MEAT, AN ANCESTRAL NUTRIENT POWERHOUSE

In recent years, there has been a lot of negative attention surrounding meat consumption, particularly red meat. Media headlines often make alarming claims about the health risks associated with red meat, but a closer examination of the evidence reveals a different story. In reality, red meat is a highly nutritious food that can contribute to overall health and well-being.

Contrary to popular belief, red meat is packed with essential vitamins, minerals, and trace elements that are crucial for human health. It is an excellent source of nutrients, such as vitamin B12, vitamin D, iron, zinc, magnesium, copper, cobalt, and more. Obtaining these vitamins and minerals from whole-food sources, like red meat, is extremely beneficial as relying solely on government-fortified processed foods does not provide sufficient intake. Let's take a closer look at some of the amazing health benefits of red meat:

- **Vitamin D:** Red meat is particularly important for individuals who have limited sun exposure or consume little oily fish. That's because it significantly contributes to your vitamin D intake. Red meat contains a vitamin D metabolite called 25-hydroxycholecalciferol, which is more easily absorbed and utilized by the body compared to other dietary forms of vitamin D. In populations with low sun exposure, consuming meat has shown protective effects against rickets, a bone disease caused by severe vitamin D deficiency. Surprisingly, consuming the same amount of vitamin D through milk does not provide the same level of protection. This suggests that the vitamin D in meat is uniquely absorbable and beneficial to the human body.

- **Iron:** Red meat is an amazing source of heme iron, a form of iron that is absorbed and utilized more efficiently by the human body compared to non-heme iron found in plants. It's interesting to note that even modest quantities of red meat can improve the absorption of non-heme iron. Non-heme iron, which is predominantly found in plant-based sources, is less readily absorbed by the body compared to heme iron, which is found in animal-based foods. However, the inclusion of red meat in the diet can significantly enhance the absorption of non-heme iron, thereby improving iron status. This synergistic effect between red meat and non-heme iron absorption highlights the importance of dietary diversity and the potential benefits of incorporating a balanced combination of iron-rich foods into the diet.

While individuals with iron overload conditions (i.e. haemochromatosis) may need to limit their intake of iron-rich foods (i.e. red meat), for the majority of the population, especially those with iron-deficiency anemia, the iron in red meat is highly beneficial. This is particularly crucial for pregnant women or those planning to conceive, as iron is extremely vital for the development of the fetal brain.

- **Other Minerals:** Red meat plays a vital role in providing essential minerals and trace elements to our body, including zinc. In the United States, where organ meats and shellfish (other rich sources of zinc) are less commonly consumed, red meat becomes an especially important source of zinc. Similarly to vitamin D and iron, the zinc present in red meat is highly bioavailable, and even small amounts of this type of zinc in the diet can enhance zinc utilization from other sources. Zinc is an essential mineral involved in numerous physiological processes, including protein and enzyme structure, as well as gene expression. Individuals following meat-free diets are at a greater risk of developing a zinc deficiency. Additionally, red meat contains significant levels of other vital micronutrients, such as magnesium, copper, cobalt, phosphorus, chromium, nickel, and selenium, which further contribute to its impressive nutrient profile.

Red Meat is Nutritionally Superior to White Meat

While some of the benefits mentioned earlier apply to both red and white meat, red meat offers distinct advantages when it comes to certain nutrients over white meat. B vitamins, vitamin D, and most trace minerals are found in comparable levels in both red and white meat. However, red meat stands out due to its significantly higher content of vitamin B12, iron, and zinc. These alone make it a nutritionally superior option to white meat.

However, the real star of red meat lies in its fatty acid profile. The fat found in red meat coming from grass-eating animals, known as ruminants, consists of roughly equal amounts of saturated and monounsaturated fats, with only a small portion of polyunsaturated fats. Interestingly, the unique digestive system of ruminants helps maintain these proportions consistently, regardless of their diet. This aspect makes red meat particularly valuable for individuals who may not have the means to afford grass-fed meat.

Even if you opt for conventionally-raised red meat, you will still be consuming a considerable amount of saturated and monounsaturated fats, which are healthier options compared to polyunsaturated fats (PUFAs).

Including red meat in your diet can provide a rich and robust nutritional source, especially regarding essential nutrients, such as vitamin B12, iron, and zinc.

Are Trans Fats in Red Meat Bad?

Trans fats have gained a reputation for being unhealthy due to their negative impact on cholesterol levels. These fats are created through an industrial process called hydrogenation, where hydrogen molecules are added to liquid vegetable oil, altering its chemical structure and turning it into solid fat. The consumption of trans fats has been linked to an increased risk of heart disease, stroke, and other health issues.

The harmful effects of trans fats are primarily attributed to their ability to raise total cholesterol levels while lowering levels of HDL (high-density lipoprotein). This imbalance in blood lipid ratios is a concern for cardiovascular health. However, it's important to note that the risks associated with trans fats extend beyond their impact on cholesterol. Conventional nutrition advice often overlooks this aspect.

Interestingly, many foods that are typically recommended on Paleo, carnivore, or other anti-inflammatory, whole-food-based diets also contain naturally occurring trans fats. These include dairy fat and meats from grass-eating animals, known as ruminants. Grass-fed animals tend to have higher levels of these naturally occurring trans fatty acids compared to grain-fed animals. For example, a grass-fed steak contains around 0.5 to 1.4 grams of trans fat per ounce (28.3 grams) of total fat.

Now, here's the crucial point: the naturally occurring trans fats found in ruminant animal products are not considered harmful to human health. In fact, they may even offer potential health benefits and contribute to the prevention of certain chronic diseases. Studies suggest that these naturally occurring trans fats have different biological effects on the body compared to industrially produced trans fats. They may possess anti-inflammatory and anti-cancer properties and could play a positive role in improving insulin sensitivity and reducing the risk of obesity-related diseases.

CLA: How is It Different From Industrial Trans Fats?

The way naturally occurring trans fats are formed is quite different from the process used to create industrial trans fats. In ruminant animals, like cows and sheep, rumen bacteria in their stomachs break down the grass they eat and produce trans-rumenic and trans-vaccenic acid as a result of digesting the polyunsaturated fats (PUFAs) present in the grass.

One specific trans-rumenic acid, called conjugated linoleic acid (CLA), is abundant in meat and dairy products from grass-fed animals, and to a lesser extent in products from grain-fed animals. Additionally, our bodies can produce CLA by converting trans-vaccenic acid from these animal products.

Chemically speaking, industrial trans fats have slightly different structures compared to the trans fats found naturally in beef and butter. Specifically, the position of the double bond in their molecular structure differs. Furthermore, CLA contains both cis- and trans-bonds, whereas most industrial trans fats consist only of trans bonds. Despite these minor differences in structure, they have significant implications for the body, as demonstrated by numerous clinical and epidemiological studies.

Unlike industrial trans fats, which have been linked to an increased risk of heart disease, cancer, and obesity, naturally occurring trans fats like CLA found in animal products are believed to have the opposite effect. Research suggests that they may actually reduce the risk of these diseases.

Health Benefits of CLA

CLA, or conjugated linoleic acid, offers several health benefits that distinguish it from industrial trans fats, particularly in relation to heart disease and atherosclerosis.

Numerous clinical and epidemiological studies have been conducted, and when these studies are analyzed collectively, they suggest that natural trans fats found in animal products do not increase the risk of heart disease.

In fact, these studies have generally shown either a reverse relationship or no association between the intake of natural trans fats and heart disease across different geographical regions.

Although there have been limited controlled clinical trials on the effects of CLA and VA (vaccenic acid) on heart disease and atherosclerosis, the existing studies also support the notion that these natural trans fats may actually reduce the risk of heart disease. Animal studies have revealed that CLA has potent antiatherogenic effects, preventing the formation of fatty streaks and plaque in the arteries of rodents by altering the metabolism of macrophage lipids. Although more research is needed in humans, it appears that consuming grass-fed dairy and meat products, which are rich in both CLA and vitamin K2, can be beneficial for preventing heart attacks.

CLA may also play a role in preventing and managing type 2 diabetes. Studies conducted on rats have demonstrated that CLA improves glucose tolerance and enhances insulin action in skeletal muscle. Furthermore, research indicates that CLA may decrease hyperinsulinemia by increasing the production of adiponectin, a hormone that enhances insulin action and improves insulin sensitivity. Epidemiological evidence supports the idea that there is an inverse association between CLA levels in adipose tissue and the risk of diabetes, further supporting the hypothesis that CLA is involved in healthy insulin regulation.

Moreover, CLA has shown potential in reducing the risk of cancer according to both experimental and case-control studies. It primarily achieves this by inhibiting the growth and metastatic spread of tumors, regulating the cell cycle, and reducing inflammation. CLA can disrupt the metabolic pathway for the synthesis of eicosanoids, which are inflammatory compounds derived from omega-6 polyunsaturated fatty acids. By doing so, it hinders the inflammatory processes that promote the development of cancer.

CLA supplements have also been marketed for their weight loss benefits. Some research suggests that CLA can help reduce body fat and promote weight loss in overweight and obese individuals. In several studies, dietary supplementation with CLA has been found to increase lean body mass, decrease body fat mass, and improve overall body composition in overweight individuals. The proposed mechanism is that CLA enhances the breakdown of body fat and reduces its storage. However, it's important to note that the reduction in body fat achieved through CLA supplementation is modest, so it may not lead to significant weight loss as some supplement advertisers like to claim. Nonetheless, incorporating dietary sources of CLA, such as grass-fed meat and dairy products (if tolerated), may support weight loss efforts.

While scientific studies provide intriguing insights into the potential health benefits of CLA, more high-quality human research is necessary to establish its precise role in human health and disease. The encouraging news is that all foods naturally containing CLA offer additional benefits, so by emphasizing the consumption of grass-fed meat and dairy products (if suitable for you), you can obtain adequate amounts of CLA.

Red Meat: A Great Source of CLA

Red meat, particularly from grass-fed sources, is an excellent natural source of CLA (conjugated linoleic acid) and VA (vaccenic acid). In fact, animal products coming from 100% grass-fed animals contain three to five times more CLA compared to those from grain-fed animals. Since CLA is found in fatty tissue, opting for fattier cuts of meat and consuming bone marrow may provide higher amounts of CLA.

It's important to note that supplementing with CLA does not offer the same potential benefits as obtaining CLA through a diet rich in CLA-containing foods (i.e. grass-fed beef, lamb, full-fat dairy products). In fact, CLA supplements can potentially be harmful. Many CLA supplements are derived from linoleic acid found in safflower oil, and studies have indicated that CLA supplementation in humans may lead to negative health effects, such as fatty liver, inflammation, dyslipidemia, and insulin resistance. Additionally, CLA supplements have not shown the same beneficial effects observed in human trials that focused on dietary intake of CLA.

This disparity may be due to the composition of synthetic CLA supplements, where 50 percent of the product consists of an unnamed isomer, which is a different fatty acid compared to the CLA and VA naturally found in red meat. It's always preferable to obtain nutrients from real whole foods rather than relying on supplements whenever possible, and the same principle applies to CLA. If your goal is to follow a diet that supports heart health and reduces the risk of cancer, it is advisable to include generous portions of grass-fed beef in your meals. Even if your doctor has (falsely) expressed concerns about it, incorporating grass-fed red meat into your diet is beneficial from a nutritive and health point of view.

Common Myths About Red Meat

There are some general misconceptions surrounding red meat that have contributed to its negative reputation. Over the years, several studies have been published that have raised concerns about the health effects of red meat.

It's important to understand that many of these studies are observational in nature, meaning they can only establish associations rather than prove causation. Observational studies have limitations, and they are susceptible to confounding variables that can impact results. Even the most skilled statisticians struggle with addressing these confounding factors.

In other words, while these studies may suggest a link between red meat consumption and certain negative health outcomes, they cannot definitively prove that red meat is the sole cause of those outcomes. It's essential to consider the overall body of scientific evidence and approach the findings of these studies with caution and critical judgment.

The "Healthy-User Bias"

One of the significant challenges with observational studies on red meat is what scientists call the "healthy-user bias." This term describes a phenomenon where individuals who adopt one behavior perceived as healthy, whether it truly is or not, tend to adopt other healthy behaviors as well. Similarly, those who engage in behaviors perceived as unhealthy are more likely to engage in other unhealthy behaviors.

When it comes to red meat, it has received negative attention in the media for many years. As a result, people who consume less red meat are also more likely to consume less of other foods that are considered unhealthy, such as refined sugar, trans fats, and processed foods. Additionally, they are more likely to make healthier lifestyle choices, such as being physically active and not smoking.

Therefore, the apparent association between red meat consumption and negative health outcomes observed in some observational studies may be influenced by these confounding factors. It becomes very challenging to determine whether the observed effects are specifically due to red meat consumption or a combination of other factors associated with healthy or unhealthy behaviors.

It's important to consider these biases and limitations when interpreting the results of observational studies. While these studies can provide valuable insights, they cannot establish a cause-and-effect relationship between red meat consumption and health outcomes.

To gain a more comprehensive understanding, it's crucial to consider a range of scientific evidence, including randomized controlled trials and systematic reviews, which provide a higher level of evidence. These types of studies can help researchers evaluate the effects of red meat consumption while controlling for confounding variables and biases.

Questionnaires Are Not a Reliable Way of Gathering Data

When it comes to gathering data about what people eat, relying on food frequency questionnaires may not be the most reliable method. These questionnaires often require individuals to recall and report their dietary intake over a specific period, which can be prone to errors and inaccuracies. It's challenging to remember every meal and food item you consumed, making it difficult to obtain precise information.

Due to these limitations, individual studies that rely on food frequency questionnaires to examine the effects of red meat consumption have their shortcomings. They may not provide conclusive evidence due to potential biases and inaccuracies in data collection. Therefore, it's important to consider the overall body of evidence rather than solely relying on individual studies to form an informed opinion about red meat's impact on human health.

Now, let's explore and debunk five common health myths associated with red meat, providing solid reasons to approach them with skepticism.

Myth 1: Red Meat Causes Heart Disease

You might have come across alarming reports about a study published in the journal *Nature* that suggested a possible link between red meat consumption and heart disease. It's natural to feel concerned after reading such information, but there's no need to rush into replacing your red meat with soy burgers just yet.

In the study, researchers previously proposed a theory involving a chemical called TMAO (trimethylamine N-oxide), which they suggested could increase the risk of heart disease. Their hypothesis was that eating red meat might raise TMAO levels in the bloodstream, potentially elevating the chances of experiencing a heart attack. At first glance, this explanation may sound reasonable.

However, it's important to note that this study and its findings are not conclusive evidence that red meat directly causes heart disease. The research merely presents a hypothesis and explores a potential mechanism. Further investigation is needed to establish a solid cause-and-effect relationship between red meat consumption, TMAO levels, and heart disease.

It's crucial to approach such studies with caution and consider the broader body of scientific evidence. Numerous factors contribute to heart disease risk, including overall dietary patterns, lifestyle choices, genetics, and other environmental factors. Simply attributing heart disease solely to red meat oversimplifies the complex nature of this condition.

The Shortfalls of the Diet-Heart Hypothesis

There is another hypothesis that has been put forth to explain the supposed link between red meat consumption and heart disease. It is known as the "diet-heart hypothesis," and you may be familiar with it, even if you haven't heard the term before. This hypothesis suggests that consuming cholesterol and saturated fat raises cholesterol levels in the blood, which in turn leads to heart disease. Over time, this theory gained widespread acceptance, and it is rarely questioned even today.

However, recent scientific research has challenged the validity of the diet-heart hypothesis. It has been revealed that dietary saturated fat and cholesterol are not associated with an increased risk of heart disease. Even if they were, high cholesterol levels in the blood may not be the direct cause of heart disease.

Unfortunately, the misguided belief that saturated fats and cholesterol are the primary drivers of heart disease led to a decades-long campaign promoting low-fat, high-carbohydrate diets. Regrettably, the consequences of this campaign were not without harm. Not only did it unnecessarily restrict people from enjoying nutrient-dense and delicious foods, like red meat, but it may have indirectly contributed to the rise of obesity, heart disease, and diabetes we witness today.

Studies have demonstrated that when saturated fat is replaced with carbohydrates, the risk of heart disease actually increases. However, this is not solely due to carbohydrates themselves, but rather the fact that a significant portion of carbs consumed in the United States come from refined grains.

The diet-heart hypothesis serves as a cautionary tale, reminding us not to hastily jump to conclusions based on limited evidence. Unfortunately, the lack of critical examination or scrutiny in popular media reports about this study suggests that caution has been disregarded.

Let's explore the reasons why we should not readily accept the conclusions of this study that suggests red meat causes heart disease.

The Epidemiological Evidence is Inconsistent

If consuming red meat leads to elevated levels of TMAO, which in turn increases the risk of heart disease, we would expect to see higher rates of heart disease in people who consume more red meat. However, the epidemiological evidence examining this question provides mixed findings.

A comprehensive meta-analysis published in Circulation by Micha et al., which analyzed data from over 1.2 million participants, found no association between the consumption of fresh, unprocessed red meat and an increased risk of coronary heart disease (CHD), stroke, or diabetes.

On the other hand, a smaller prospective study involving approximately 121,000 participants from the Nurses' Health Study and Health Professionals Follow-up Study did find an association between red meat consumption (both fresh and processed) and total mortality, cardiovascular disease (CVD), and cancer. If eating meat indeed increases the risk of heart disease, we would expect lower rates of heart disease in vegans and vegetarians.

Early studies initially suggested this to be true, but later, better-controlled studies indicated otherwise. The early studies were flawed in design and influenced by confounding factors. For example, on average, vegetarians tend to be more health-conscious than the general population, engaging in more exercise and less smoking, among other factors that could explain their longevity.

Newer, higher-quality studies that have attempted to account for these confounding factors have not found any survival advantage in vegetarians. One study compared the mortality rates of both vegetarians and omnivores who shopped at health food stores with those of the general population. The study found that both vegetarians and omnivores in the health food store group lived longer than people in the general population.

These findings suggest that consuming meat as part of a healthy diet does not have the same effects as consuming meat within an unhealthy diet. A large-scale study conducted in the United Kingdom in 2003, involving over 65,000 subjects, supported these results, as no difference in mortality was observed between vegetarians and omnivores.

Collectively, these data do not provide strong evidence of a significant relationship between red meat consumption and heart disease. It is important to remember that epidemiological evidence, as mentioned earlier, does not establish causality. Even if there is indeed an association between red meat intake and a higher risk of CVD or any other health problem, such studies do not prove that red meat is the cause of the problem.

The Healthy-User Bias Strikes Again

The healthy-user bias greatly complicates our ability to establish a causal relationship from epidemiological findings. Let's consider a hypothetical study that suggests consuming processed meats, such as bacon and hot dogs, increases the risk of heart disease.

Now, let's imagine that the healthy-user bias comes into play, as predicted. Individuals who consume more bacon and hot dogs might also have a higher intake of refined flour (found in hot dog and hamburger buns), sugar, and industrial seed oils. Additionally, they may consume fewer fresh fruits, vegetables, and soluble fiber. They may also engage in habits, such as increased alcohol consumption, smoking, and reduced physical activity. Essentially, their overall self-care and lifestyle choices may be suboptimal.

In light of these factors, how can we determine whether it is specifically the processed meat that is responsible for the increased risk of heart disease, or if it is a combination of these other factors along with the processed meat? The truth is, we don't have a definitive answer. Well-designed studies make efforts to control for some of these confounding factors, but it is inevitable that some factors may go uncontrolled. One critical confounding factor that is typically not addressed is the gut microbiome, which refers to the community of microorganisms living in our digestive system.

Considering all these complexities, it becomes challenging to establish a direct link between processed meat consumption and heart disease, separate from the influence of other lifestyle and dietary factors. The presence of the healthy-user bias and uncontrolled confounding factors makes it difficult to draw definitive conclusions from observational studies alone.

As said, one crucial factor that oftentimes goes unaccounted for in studies is the gut microbiome, which refers to the diverse community of microorganisms residing in our digestive system. These microscopic organisms play a vital role in our health, influencing various aspects of our physiology, metabolism, immune function, and even mental well-being.

The gut microbiome is highly individualized, shaped by factors such as genetics, diet, lifestyle, and exposure to environmental influences. It has the ability to break down and interact with the foods we consume, including processed meats. Different individuals have distinct gut microbiome compositions, which can affect how their bodies respond to specific dietary components.

When it comes to studying the impact of processed meat on health, researchers rarely account for the diversity and activity of the gut microbiome. This means that the potential influence of these microorganisms on the relationship between processed meat consumption and heart disease is often overlooked or not fully understood.

Considering the significant role of the gut microbiome in our overall health and its potential to interact with the foods we eat, it is an important factor to consider when examining the complex relationship between diet and chronic disease. Further research is needed to explore how the gut microbiome may influence the effects of processed meat consumption on heart health and other aspects of human health.

The Gut Microbiome: A Key Regulator of Human Health

Mounting evidence suggests that the composition of bacteria in our gut, known as the gut microbiome, plays a crucial role in determining our overall health and well-being. When the balance of healthy and unhealthy bacteria in the gut is disrupted, it can lead to various health issues, including skin problems, depression, anxiety, autoimmune conditions, and even hair loss.

The study we're discussing here focused on the production of a compound called TMAO, which has been associated with red meat consumption. The researchers found that individuals who eat red meat produce TMAO, while vegans and vegetarians who have avoided meat for a year or longer do not. The researchers concluded that red meat alters the gut flora in a way that promotes TMAO production. However, there's a more plausible explanation: red meat eaters may engage in other unhealthy behaviors that disrupt the balance of their gut bacteria, leading to TMAO production.

These unhealthy behaviors may include consuming fewer fruits and vegetables, lower intake of soluble fiber, and higher consumption of processed and refined foods, like flour, sugar, and seed oils. Research has shown that these behaviors are more common among the average red meat eater and have been linked to unfavorable changes in the gut microbiota. In other words, the issue may not lie with red meat itself, but rather with the state of the gut bacteria.

Supporting this notion, the study found that red meat eaters did not produce TMAO after receiving a course of antibiotics, which can disrupt the gut microbiome. Additionally, evidence suggests that a compromised intestinal barrier, which occurs in conditions like dysbiosis and SIBO, may increase the risk of heart disease by raising the number of harmful LDL particles in the bloodstream.

Currently, the available evidence indicates that the effects of eating meat may differ depending on the overall quality of one's diet. This study is likely another example of this phenomenon. To determine whether red meat truly causes changes in the gut flora that increase TMAO production, further research is needed. One way to investigate this connection would be to conduct a study with two groups:

1. A group following a Paleo diet rich in fruits, vegetables, soluble fiber, and red meat.

2. Another group adhering to a vegan/vegetarian diet with equivalent amounts of plant-based foods, but no meat.

By comparing the TMAO levels between these two groups, stronger evidence could be obtained to support or challenge the hypothesis that red meat consumption directly influences TMAO production. These types of studies have the potential to deepen our understanding of the intricate interplay between diet, gut bacteria composition, and its impact on health outcomes. By examining different dietary patterns and their effects on gut microbiota, we can gain valuable insights into how our food choices shape the complex relationship between our gut microbiome and overall well-being.

The TMAO Puzzle: More Questions Than Answers

The connection between TMAO production, red meat consumption, and the risk of heart disease is not as straightforward as the authors of the study suggest. The study in question presented data from two different studies: one involving humans and another involving mice.

The human study was quite limited, comparing only a single vegan person who was convinced to eat a steak with five supposed representative meat-eaters. With a sample size of just six individuals, with only one in the vegan group, it's challenging to draw definitive conclusions from such a small study.

The mouse study used a carnitine supplement to stimulate TMAO production. While it is known that free carnitine can increase TMAO levels, previous studies have not shown that carnitine-rich foods like red meat directly lead to elevated TMAO levels. In fact, a 1999 study testing 46 different foods, including red meat, found that only seafood raised TMAO levels. This is expected since seafood naturally contains trimethylamine, a precursor to TMAO. So, should we be concerned about seafood causing heart attacks?

Another important question to consider is whether there are alternative explanations for elevated TMAO levels in meat or seafood eaters (assuming we observe such elevations in a broader sample of meat-eaters, which is not supported by at least one previous study).

According to a 2011 article on TMAO in a different context, elevated TMAO levels could be attributed to dietary trimethylamine or TMAO from seafood. However, they could also be influenced by impaired excretion in the urine or enhanced conversion of trimethylamine to TMAO in the liver. This conversion is carried out by an enzyme called Fmo3, primarily in the liver. Genetic variations affecting this enzyme's activity exist and some of them are specific to certain ethnic groups. This enzyme also processes various drugs used to treat different health conditions. Iron or salt overload can also impact its activity. Therefore, elevated TMAO levels might be a marker for ethnicity, drug exposure, genetically determined drug response, or other health conditions.

Even if meat eaters indeed have higher TMAO levels compared to vegans and vegetarians, we still lack evidence to establish a direct cause-and-effect relationship between TMAO and cardiovascular disease (CVD). Once again, the link between cholesterol, saturated fat, and heart disease should serve as a reminder not to hastily jump to conclusions that deprive people of healthy, nutrient-dense foods. It is nearly impossible to control for all potential confounding factors, and the study we're discussing further highlights this challenge.

Myth 2: Eating Red Meat Causes Cancer

Every year, there seems to be an onslaught from the medical community suggesting that red meat causes cancer. But what does the research truly reveal about the connection between red meat and cancer? The World Health Organization (WHO) classified processed meats, like bacon and sausage, as "group 1 carcinogens," putting them in the same category as substances known to cause cancer, such as tobacco, asbestos, alcohol, and arsenic. Fresh red meat was placed in the "group 2A" category, suggesting it is "probably carcinogenic" to humans. This argument has been around for at least 40 years, with scientists speculating about the link between animal product consumption and cancer since 1975.

However, the evidence supporting this claim is not as strong as its proponents make it out to be. Let's look at a critical review published in the esteemed scientific journal *Obesity Reviews* in 2010. The authors examined 35 studies that claimed an association between red meat and cancer and identified numerous issues. Here are some key findings and their implications:

• The association between red meat consumption and colorectal cancer is generally weak and often statistically insignificant. Comparing bacon to cigarettes is misleading because the evidence does not support a strong link between red meat and cancer. In fact, some studies even show a decrease in cancer rates among people who consume more red meat.

- Different studies report varying rates of cancer in different parts of the intestinal tract and among men and women. For example, some studies found an inverse relationship between red meat intake and colon cancer (meaning more red meat consumption was associated with less colon cancer), while a positive relationship was observed with rectal cancer. These inconsistent findings cast doubt on a direct causal relationship between red meat and cancer.

- The studies linking red meat and cancer often fail to account for other dietary and lifestyle factors, such as a Western-style diet, high intake of refined sugars and alcohol, low intake of fruits, vegetables, and fiber, low physical activity, high smoking prevalence, and high body mass index (BMI). These factors can confound the results and introduce bias.

In an ideal scenario, a randomized controlled trial would be conducted to definitively determine whether red meat causes cancer. However, this is impractical due to the long timeframe required for cancer development and the cost involved. As a result, we rely on observational studies, which only demonstrate an association between variables, but do not prove causality. Observational studies have limitations, especially the presence of the healthy-user bias. Individuals who consume more red meat in these studies also tend to engage in other unhealthy behaviors like smoking, excessive alcohol consumption, and a poor overall diet. It's worth noting that many Americans who eat red meat also consume it alongside refined carbohydrates and unhealthy fats. This raises the question: Is it the red meat itself or the combined effects of other unhealthy foods that contribute to the increased cancer risk? While researchers strive to minimize the influence of confounding factors, it is challenging to completely eliminate them in observational studies. Therefore, the evidence linking red meat to cancer remains inconclusive, and it is crucial to interpret the results with caution.

Gut Microbiome's Role in Cancer Pathophysiology

What's more, certain factors are likely to play a significant role in the relationship between any food that we eat and cancer, but they have never been adequately controlled for in any study. One of these factors is the gut microbiome, the collection of microorganisms in our digestive system. Research has indicated that the composition of the gut microbiota can directly influence how dietary factors affect our risk of developing cancer.

For instance, certain bacteria like *Streptococcus bovis*, *Bacteroides*, *Fusobacterium*, *Clostridia*, and *Helicobacter pylori* have been associated with tumor development, while others like *Lactobacillus acidophilus*, *L. plantarum*, and *Bifidobacterium longum* have been found to inhibit colon cancer formation. Studies have also observed differences in the abundance of specific bacterial species between populations at high and low risk of colon cancer.

A recent study compared the gut microbiota of 60 patients with colorectal cancer to that of 119 healthy individuals. The cancer patients showed significant increases in the levels of *Bacteroides/Prevotella* (potentially harmful bacterial species) compared to the control group. This difference remained consistent regardless of patient characteristics like age, body mass index (BMI), family history of cancer, tumor size or location, or disease stage. In other words, an individual with an imbalanced or compromised microbiome may be at higher risk of cancer if they consume high amounts of fresh or processed red meat. However, someone with a normal and healthy microbiome may not face the same risk.

This highlights the importance of considering the complex interplay between our gut microbiota and dietary factors when evaluating the potential links between red meat and cancer. Future research will likely delve further into understanding how our gut health influences the impact of specific foods on cancer risk.

Drawing Inaccurate Conclusions From Observational Studies

Observational studies have their uses in generating ideas and identifying general patterns. However, they have limitations, including their inability to account for crucial differences among study participants.

Let's consider two individuals as an example:

- **Person A:** Follows a Standard American Diet (SAD), leads a sedentary lifestyle, and has an imbalanced gut microbiome.

- **Person B:** Follows a Paleo-type diet, exercises regularly, and maintains a healthy gut microbiome.

In observational studies investigating the relationship between red meat and cancer, the majority (at least 95 percent or more) of red meat eaters included in typical studies belong to the first category (Person A).

If a study concludes that there is a link between red meat and cancer, the 5 percent of participants who follow a healthy diet, engage in regular exercise, and have a healthy gut—making them less likely to experience the same negative effects from consuming red meat—are grouped together with the other 95 percent.

To put it differently, considering what we already know about the impact of diet, lifestyle, and the microbiome on cancer risk, it should be evident that someone following a Paleo-type diet and lifestyle will not have the same cancer risk as someone following a Standard American Diet (SAD) and lifestyle, even if they consume an equivalent amount of red meat. Yet, these two groups are consistently grouped together in studies and media reports. This presents a significant problem in research that has not been adequately addressed.

Essentially, when interpreting observational studies, it is important to recognize that the data might not distinguish between individuals with vastly different lifestyles, diets, and gut health statuses. Consequently, the reported associations between red meat and cancer may not be accurately representative of the effects on all individuals consuming red meat.

The Red Meat-Cancer Connection: Final Thoughts

Even if we consider the World Health Organization's report without questioning its validity, it's important to understand the actual impact of eating cured and processed meats on cancer risk. According to an article in *The Guardian*, consuming cured and processed meats would result in approximately three additional cases of bowel cancer per 100,000 adults. This means that your chances of developing bowel cancer from eating these meats are roughly 1 in 33,000. This is significantly different from the increased risk associated with smoking cigarettes, which the WHO now places in the same category as eating bacon and salami. As Professor Ian Johnson of the Quadram Institute has pointed out in the past, comparing the adverse effects of bacon and sausages on bowel cancer risk to the dangers of tobacco smoke is highly inappropriate. Tobacco smoke contains known chemical carcinogens and raises the risk of lung cancer in smokers by approximately twentyfold (2000%).

Furthermore, the WHO report categorized 940 other agents, along with red meat, as potential carcinogens. Betsy Booren, the vice president of scientific affairs for the North American Meat Institute, offered some perspective in The Guardian article. She highlighted that the International Agency for Research on Cancer (IARC) suggests you can enjoy activities like yoga, but should avoid breathing air (considered a class 1 carcinogen), sitting near a sun-filled window (class 1), applying aloe vera after sunburn (class 2B), drinking wine or coffee (class 1 and class 2B), or eating grilled food (class 2A). Additionally, if you work as a hairdresser or do shift work, both are classified as class 2A carcinogens, according to the IARC.

Based on current research findings, it is highly unlikely that moderate consumption of cured or processed meat poses a significant health risk, especially if you are taking other positive steps, such as nurturing your gut microbiome, consuming nutrient-dense whole foods, and engaging in regular exercise.

There is even less evidence suggesting that we should limit our consumption of fresh red meat, particularly when it is prepared using gentle cooking methods rather than being charred. Additionally, when we consume other parts of the animal, apart from muscle meat, such as organs, glands, and connective tissues, we benefit from various nutrients and anti-inflammatory compounds they contain, such as specific amino acids, essential fatty acids, vitamins, minerals, trace elements, and bioactive compounds. These dietary components play a pivotal role in promoting overall health and well-being.

For instance, organ meats like liver are nutrient powerhouses, providing an abundant supply of vitamins A, D, E, K, B vitamins, and essential minerals such as iron, zinc, and copper. These nutrients are vital for optimal organ function, immune support, and energy production.

Glands, such as the adrenal and thyroid glands, offer a unique profile of compounds that support hormonal balance and metabolic health. The inclusion of these glandular tissues in our diet can help regulate stress responses, improve thyroid function, and enhance overall endocrine health.

Connective tissue, rich in collagen and gelatin, provides essential building blocks for maintaining healthy joints, tendons, ligaments, and skin. Consuming connective tissue supports our body's own collagen synthesis, promoting joint flexibility, reducing inflammation, and promoting skin elasticity and health.

Furthermore, the consumption of these animal parts introduces specific amino acids, such as glycine, proline, and glutamine, which are integral for gut health, immune function, and tissue repair. These amino acids also possess anti-inflammatory properties that can help modulate immune responses and reduce systemic inflammation.

By embracing the consumption of various parts of the animal, we not only expand our nutrient intake but also tap into a vast array of bioactive compounds that support our overall health and well-being. It is important to view the animal, no matter what it is (i.e. cow, sheep, bison, buffalo, etc) as a whole and appreciate the diverse nutritional and functional benefits that each one of its parts offers.

Myth 3: Red Meat Is Inflammatory

Contrary to popular belief, red meat can be a very healthy dietary choice due to its exceptional nutritional profile and favorable fatty acid composition. However, concerns have been raised about certain components in red meat that are commonly associated with inflammation. Are these concerns valid, or is it another case of unnecessary fear-mongering? Let's take a closer look.

Two controlled trials have investigated the effects of increased red meat consumption on inflammation markers, and both studies found no evidence that red meat raises these markers. In fact, one study even concluded that replacing carbohydrates with red meat in the diet of non-anemic individuals actually reduced inflammation markers. Another study involving anemic women showed that inflammation markers on a high-red-meat diet were not significantly different from those on a diet high in oily fish.

This evidence suggests that red meat is not inherently more inflammatory than other types of meat for most people and may even be less inflammatory than dietary carbohydrates. However, it's worth noting that red meat does contain certain compounds that are often blamed for inducing inflammation.

Neu5Gc

One compound in red meat called Neu5Gc has raised concerns regarding inflammation. Neu5Gc is a type of signalling molecule found in mammalian cells. Humans lost the ability to produce Neu5Gc millions of years ago, but we still incorporate it into our tissues when we consume red meat. Some researchers have suggested that the interaction between Neu5Gc and anti-Neu5Gc antibodies in our bodies may lead to chronic inflammation and diseases like cancer. However, it's important to highlight that this hypothesis is far from proven, as research in this area is still in its early stages. Most studies acknowledge that any role of Neu5Gc in chronic inflammation is speculative at this point.

Arachidonic Acid (AA)

Arachidonic acid (AA), found primarily in animal-based foods, such as meat, eggs, and dairy products, is often cited as a source of inflammation. However, AA plays a crucial role in the body's inflammatory response and is necessary for growth and repair. The interplay between AA and other fatty acids is complex, and an imbalance in these fats can have undesirable effects.

Interestingly, epidemiological studies have shown that higher levels of both AA and long-chain omega-3 fatty acids are associated with lower levels of inflammatory markers. Clinical studies have also demonstrated that adding substantial amounts of AA to the diet has no significant effect on inflammatory cytokine production in the body.

It's worth noting that our Paleolithic ancestors consumed twice as much AA as the average modern American today without suffering from chronic inflammatory diseases.

Charred Meat and Cancer

Concerns have been raised about compounds produced when meat is cooked, such as advanced glycation end products (AGEs), heterocyclic amines (HAs), and polycyclic aromatic hydrocarbons (PAHs). While these compounds can potentially cause cancer in animal models, it's important to remember that they are present in all types of meat, not just red meat.

Limiting exposure to these compounds is wise, especially HAs and PAHs, which are formed when meat is cooked using high-heat or dry-cooking methods. However, it's interesting to note that the highest levels of PAHs are found in charred meats cooked over an open flame.

Furthermore, dietary AGEs, which may also contribute to inflammation, are present in both cooked and uncooked meat but do not necessarily pose a significant concern for most people.

To minimize the formation of these compounds, favor wet or low-heat cooking methods for meat. Alternatively, using an acidic marinade can significantly reduce the formation of these compounds while enhancing flavor.

Marinating meat for as little as one hour can cut AGE formation by over half, and acidic marinades can reduce HA formation by up to 90 percent.

Red Meat and Inflammation: Final Thoughts

In summary, there is no solid evidence to suggest that red meat is more inflammatory than other types of meat. In fact, some evidence indicates that it may be less inflammatory. Individual intolerances to red meat can cause inflammation in some people, but for most individuals, there is no reason to restrict red meat based on inflammation concerns.

Furthermore, the worries about AGEs in meat are likely unfounded, and meat-eaters may even have lesser plasma levels of AGEs than non-meat-eaters. Any concerns regarding compounds produced during meat cooking can be minimized by favoring wet or low-heat cooking methods or by using acidic marinades when high-heat methods are desired.

It's essential to consider that red meat has been a part of the human diet for a significant portion of our evolutionary history and remains a key dietary component in many healthy cultures around the world. For instance, the Maasai people in East Africa traditionally consume a diet consisting mostly of red meat (specifically, cows, goats, and sheep), calf blood, and raw milk, all of which are significant sources of Neu5Gc, yet they have been free from modern inflammatory diseases.

If Neu5Gc truly caused significant inflammation, the Maasai would have experienced its effects.

Myth 4: Red Meat Causes Kidney Disease in Healthy People

The relationship between red meat consumption and kidney disease in healthy individuals has been a subject of scientific investigation. While high-protein diets have been associated with potential harm for individuals with existing kidney disease, it is crucial to emphasize that a high-protein diet does not directly cause kidney disease in healthy individuals. To fully understand this concept, it is necessary to explore the mechanisms involved and examine the scientific evidence.

One common misconception is that consuming more protein places excessive strain on the kidneys. The kidneys play a vital role in metabolizing and excreting nitrogen byproducts from protein digestion. The body has intrinsic mechanisms to regulate protein consumption, driven by complex physiological processes and mechanisms beyond conscious control.

High-protein diets have been observed to induce measurable changes in kidney function. These changes include increases in glomerular filtration rate (GFR), often referred to as "hyperfiltration," as well as an increase in the size and volume of glomeruli, which are the functional filtration units of the kidneys. However, these changes are not necessarily indicative of kidney stress or damage. Instead, they are viewed as normal adaptive responses of the kidneys to the increased protein load.

For instance, during pregnancy, GFR significantly increases as an adaptive response to support the increased metabolic demands of the mom and baby. Despite this increase in GFR, there is no corresponding increase in the risk of kidney disease during pregnancy. Another compelling example is observed in individuals who have voluntarily donated one of their kidneys. Following donation, the remaining kidney experiences an increase in GFR as an adaptive response, and this elevated GFR persists over time. Importantly, scientific studies have consistently shown that these individuals do not have a higher risk of developing kidney disease, even years after donation.

A comprehensive review of published research on high-protein diets and kidney disease concluded that while high-protein diets can be harmful to individuals with pre-existing kidney disease, they do not cause harm to the kidneys in healthy individuals. Furthermore, subsequent studies investigating the effects of high-protein diets on renal function in healthy individuals have consistently supported this conclusion. It is worth noting that individual variations in kidney function and health should also be considered. In some rare cases, individuals with certain genetic or pre-existing conditions may have a higher sensitivity to dietary protein intake. However, these cases are exceptional and do not reflect the typical response of healthy individuals.

Overall, the belief that red meat consumption and high-protein diets cause kidney disease in healthy individuals is not supported by scientific evidence. While high-protein diets can have adverse effects on individuals with pre-existing kidney disease, the changes in kidney function observed in response to high-protein diets in healthy individuals are considered normal adaptations rather than indications of kidney disease. Extensive research and reviews have consistently demonstrated that high-protein diets do not harm the kidneys in healthy individuals.

Myth 5: Red Meat Causes Gout

Gout, a form of inflammatory arthritis, is characterized by high levels of uric acid in the blood, leading to the formation of crystal deposits in joints and surrounding tissues, particularly in the feet and big toe joint. In the past, gout was associated with affluent individuals who could afford indulgent foods, such as meat, sugar, and alcohol. Uric acid is a byproduct of purine metabolism, which is found in varying levels in all foods, including red meat, which is commonly emphasized in nutrient-dense, ancestral diets.

Patients with gout are often advised to reduce or eliminate purine-rich foods to manage uric acid production and alleviate gout symptoms. Research has indeed confirmed the association between high purine intake and acute gout attacks, suggesting that individuals diagnosed with gout may benefit from reducing their consumption of purine-rich foods. This raises the question of whether red meat, being nutrient-dense and purine-rich, is a risk factor for gout, especially among those following meat-heavy diets, such as Paleo, keto, or carnivore.

While a high purine intake is associated with gout attacks in individuals with hyperuricemia (elevated uric acid levels in the blood), it is important to note that purine intake alone is not sufficient to trigger these attacks. Interestingly, uric acid levels can decrease during gout attacks, sometimes falling within the normal range. Another factor linked to gout flares is an increase in inflammatory markers, like C-reactive protein (CRP) and interleukin-6 (IL-6), which are elevated during various inflammatory conditions. These cytokines are found in higher levels in the joint fluid and serum of patients with acute gouty arthritis.

This suggests that systemic inflammation plays a significant role in the likelihood of experiencing gout flares, and diet is a major influencer of inflammation. Although red meat is high in purines, it also contains higher levels of omega-3 fatty acids and lower levels of omega-6 fatty acids compared to grain-fed meat. The balance between omega-3s and omega-6s in the diet has a direct impact on the inflammatory status of the body. A diet rich in long-chain omega-3 fats, like EPA and DHA, can reduce systemic inflammation and potentially lower the risk of forming uric acid crystals that cause joint pain.

Furthermore, fructose, when consumed in excessive amounts, can contribute to the development of gout. Studies have shown that a high fructose intake may lead to abnormalities associated with metabolic syndrome, including elevated triglycerides due to increased uric acid production. Research has confirmed that fructose ingestion raises uric acid levels by promoting excess uric acid production and reducing its excretion in the urine. While a certain level of uric acid in the blood is normal and provides antioxidant protection, excessive uric acid acts as a pro-oxidant (the opposite effect to antioxidants) and is the primary causative factor for gout. Some researchers even suggest that elevated uric acid levels are a significant factor in the development of insulin resistance and metabolic disorders. Thus, avoiding excessive fructose consumption from sources like high-fructose corn syrup (HFCS) and table sugar can lower the risk of gout.

It is worth considering the epidemiological correlation between red meat and gout. Many conventional medical professionals associate red meat consumption with a higher risk of gout due to its association with the "Western diet pattern," which typically includes low fruit and vegetable intake and high consumption of sugar, vegetable oils, sweetened beverages, refined grains, and processed meats. When studying modern cultures, it becomes challenging for epidemiologists to isolate the effects of meat consumption from this overall dietary pattern. Additionally, most big meat consumers often exhibit other unhealthy habits and tend to be more overweight, which can confound the results of epidemiological studies. However, this does not account for health-conscious individuals who follow Paleo or carnivore diets and adopt a more mindful approach to their nutrition. These individuals actively avoid high-fructose corn syrup, excessive omega-6 fatty acids, and other inflammatory foods, like refined grains. They also tend to avoid heavy alcohol consumption and smoking.

It is important to emphasize that a diet rich in nutrient-dense foods, such as grass-fed red meat, liver, shellfish, and fatty ocean fish does not increase the risk of developing gout. On the contrary, it is the consumption of common components of the Standard American Diet (SAD) that pose a greater risk for gout. These include sugar-sweetened beverages, industrial seed and vegetable oils, refined carbohydrates, and excessive alcohol consumption, especially beer.

While it is understandable why some may associate red meat with gout due to its purine content, the comprehensive understanding of gout development suggests that other factors, such as systemic inflammation and fructose intake, play a more significant role. A well-balanced, anti-inflammatory diet like the Paleo diet, which focuses on nutrient-dense whole foods and avoids pro-inflammatory substances, may actually contribute to reducing the risk of gout.

Finally, it is crucial to note that individual responses to dietary factors can vary, and some individuals with specific medical conditions or genetic predispositions may be more sensitive to certain dietary components.

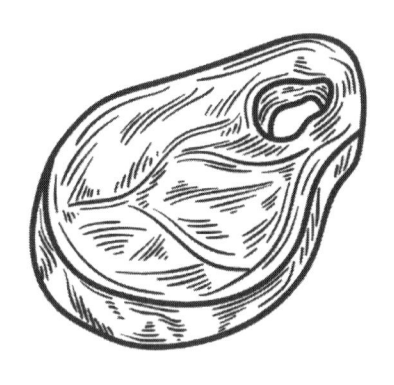

CHAPTER 3: KETO VS. CARNIVORE

Exploring the Ketogenic Diet

In recent years, the ketogenic diet has gained significant attention and popularity as a potential solution for weight loss, improved metabolic health, reduced inflammation, and increased energy levels. Also known as the keto diet, this low-carbohydrate, moderate-protein, and high-fat dietary approach has garnered interest from individuals seeking a new approach to nutrition and overall wellness.

Understanding the Ketogenic Diet

The ketogenic diet is characterized by its unique macronutrient composition. It involves a significant reduction in carbohydrate intake, typically to less than 50 grams per day, and an increase in dietary fat consumption. The restriction of carbohydrates forces the body to enter a metabolic state called ketosis, where it primarily relies on fat for energy production instead of carbohydrates. This shift in metabolism and substrate utilization has various implications for the body and can lead to several potential benefits. Let's explore some of them.

Benefits of the Ketogenic Diet

The ketogenic diet comes with several potential benefits, including:

1. Weight Loss: One of the primary reasons individuals choose the ketogenic diet is its potential for weight loss. By limiting carbohydrates, the body depletes its glycogen stores and begins to burn stored fat as its primary source of fuel. This can result in substantial weight loss, especially in combination with a calorie deficit.

2. Improved Insulin Sensitivity: The ketogenic diet has been found to enhance insulin sensitivity, which is crucial for individuals with type 2 diabetes or metabolic syndrome. By reducing carbohydrate intake, blood sugar levels are finally able to stabilize, and the body becomes more efficient at utilizing the hormone insulin.

3. Enhanced Mental Clarity and Focus: Many proponents of the ketogenic diet claim improved mental clarity and focus as additional benefits of the diet. Some studies suggest that ketones, produced during ketosis, serve as an alternative fuel source for the brain and can contribute to improved cognitive performance.

4. Reduced Inflammation: Chronic inflammation is associated with various health conditions, including heart disease, diabetes, and certain types of cancers. The ketogenic diet has shown great potential in reducing inflammation markers, such as C-reactive protein (CRP) and interleukin-6 (IL-6), which can contribute to improved overall health.

5. Increased Energy Levels: By utilizing fat as the primary energy source, individuals on the ketogenic diet often report higher and steadier energy levels, and reduced energy crashes commonly associated with carbohydrate-rich diets.

Potential Risks and Considerations

While the ketogenic diet offers many health benefits, it is important to acknowledge some potential risks and considerations associated with this dietary approach:

1. Nutrient Deficiencies

The strict limitations on carbohydrate intake in the ketogenic diet can potentially lead to inadequate consumption of certain essential nutrients. Carbohydrate-rich foods like fruits, whole grains, and legumes are excellent sources of vitamins, minerals, and dietary fiber. Therefore, individuals following a ketogenic diet should be mindful of their nutrient intake to avoid potential deficiencies.

One particular group of nutrients that may be affected by the ketogenic diet is water-soluble vitamins, such as vitamin C and B-complex vitamins. These vitamins are commonly found in fruits, vegetables, and whole grains, which are restricted or minimized in the ketogenic diet. Thus, keto followers should consider incorporating alternative sources of these vitamins, such as low-carbohydrate vegetables or even specific supplements, to maintain optimal levels.

Minerals and trace elements like potassium, magnesium, and selenium may also be at risk of deficiency due to the limited intake of certain foods. Potassium, for instance, is abundant in fruits and starchy vegetables (i.e. white potatoes) that are typically restricted in the ketogenic diet. Including low-carbohydrate sources of these minerals, such as avocados, nuts, and seeds, can help address potential deficiencies.

Moreover, dietary fiber, which is crucial for maintaining digestive health and preventing constipation, is primarily found in carbohydrate-rich foods like whole grains, legumes, and certain fruits. Since the ketogenic diet significantly restricts these foods, individuals may face challenges in meeting their daily fiber requirements. To counter this, incorporating low-carbohydrate, fiber-rich foods such as leafy greens, broccoli, and flaxseeds can support bowel regularity and overall digestive health.

To ensure nutritional needs are adequately met while following a ketogenic diet, careful meal planning is essential. By including a diverse range of low-carbohydrate, nutrient-dense foods, keto followers can help reduce the risk of any deficiencies.

2. Keto Flu

When embarking on the ketogenic diet, it's not uncommon for individuals to experience a temporary set of symptoms known as the "keto flu." This phase occurs during the initial transition as the body adapts to using fat as its primary fuel source instead of carbohydrates. While not everyone experiences these symptoms, they can include fatigue, headaches, irritability, nausea, dizziness, brain fog, and muscle cramps.

The keto flu is thought to arise due to several factors. Firstly, as carbohydrate intake is significantly reduced, the body's glycogen stores become depleted. Glycogen is the stored form of glucose in the body and serves as a readily available energy source. As glycogen levels drop, the body needs to adapt to using alternative fuel sources, such as ketones derived from fat metabolism.

During this transition, the body may experience changes in electrolyte balance, particularly with sodium, potassium, and magnesium. Reduced carbohydrate intake can affect insulin levels, leading to increased excretion of these electrolytes through urine. Consequently, electrolyte imbalances can contribute to symptoms like fatigue, headaches, and muscle cramps.

Fortunately, the keto flu is typically temporary and self-resolving as the body adjusts to the ketogenic state. To alleviate these symptoms and support the transition, individuals can take several measures. Increasing water intake can help maintain hydration and support electrolyte balance. Consuming foods rich in electrolytes, such as leafy greens, nuts, and seeds, can provide additional support.

Supplementing with electrolytes, particularly sodium, potassium, and magnesium, may be beneficial during the initial stages of the ketogenic diet. This can be achieved through specific electrolyte supplements or by adding salt to foods and incorporating foods naturally high in these minerals.

Additionally, ensuring adequate rest, managing stress levels, and gradually easing into the ketogenic diet rather than making sudden drastic changes can help minimize the severity of keto flu symptoms.

3. Cholesterol and Heart Health

The influence of the ketogenic diet on cholesterol levels has been a topic of ongoing discussion and research. Some studies have indicated that following a ketogenic diet may lead to an increase in LDL cholesterol, which is commonly referred to as "bad" cholesterol. However, it is crucial to consider the broader context of the diet's impact on overall cholesterol profile, including HDL ("good" cholesterol) and triglyceride levels.

While the increase in LDL cholesterol may raise some concerns, it's worth noting that the ketogenic diet has been shown to have favorable effects on other aspects of the cholesterol profile. Research suggests that HDL cholesterol, which is associated with a reduced risk of heart disease, tends to increase or remain unchanged on a ketogenic diet. Additionally, triglyceride levels, another important marker of heart health, typically decrease or show improvement with keto.

Furthermore, the focus of the ketogenic diet on reducing carbohydrate intake and increasing consumption of healthy fats may contribute to a shift in cholesterol particle size. Keto has been found to promote the formation of larger, less dense LDL particles, which are considered less atherogenic, meaning they are less likely to contribute to the development of plaque in arteries.

It's important to recognize that individual responses to the ketogenic diet can vary, and the impact on cholesterol levels may differ between individuals. Factors such as genetics, baseline cholesterol levels, and overall metabolic health can influence how an individual's cholesterol profile responds to the diet.

Regular monitoring of cholesterol levels, particularly when adopting significant dietary changes, is generally recommended to assess individual responses and ensure overall cardiovascular health.

4. Sustainability and Social Implications

Sustaining the ketogenic diet over the long term can pose certain challenges due to its restrictive nature, particularly in terms of limiting carbohydrate-rich foods. Many commonly consumed staple foods, such as grains, legumes, fruits, and starchy vegetables, are restricted or completely eliminated, which can make it more difficult to adhere to the diet and potentially lead to feelings of deprivation or monotony in food choices.

Furthermore, following a ketogenic diet may require careful planning and consideration in social situations and dining out. The emphasis on low-carbohydrate, high-fat foods can differ significantly from typical meals shared with friends, family, or colleagues. Attending social gatherings or restaurants may involve navigating menu options or communicating specific dietary needs, which can be challenging or uncomfortable for some individuals.

The strict adherence to the ketogenic diet may also limit the diversity of food sources and potentially lead to a higher environmental impact. Carbohydrate-rich foods like fruits, whole grains, and legumes are often associated with sustainable agricultural practices and can contribute to a varied and environmentally friendly diet. By restricting these food groups, the ketogenic diet may not align with sustainable food choices, depending on the sourcing and environmental impact of the high-fat foods that replace them.

It is important to note that sustainability and social implications are complex topics that extend beyond the dietary aspect alone. Factors such as cultural traditions, personal values, and individual health goals can influence an individual's decision to follow a particular diet, including the ketogenic diet.

To address the challenges related to sustainability and social implications, individuals following a ketogenic diet may consider incorporating environmentally conscious choices within the framework of the diet. This can include selecting locally sourced and sustainably produced high-fat foods, prioritizing quality animal products from ethical sources, and ensuring overall dietary diversity to support nutritional needs.

Open communication with friends, family, and social circles about dietary choices can also help navigate social situations and minimize potential discomfort.

Implementing the Ketogenic Diet

Adopting the ketogenic diet requires careful planning and understanding of macronutrient ratios. To achieve and sustain ketosis, individuals must prioritize high-fat foods such as avocados, nuts, seeds, fatty cuts of meat, fatty fish, and healthy oils. Carbohydrate sources should primarily come from non-starchy vegetables while limiting the intake of sugary foods, grains, and starchy vegetables.

Practical Tips for Implementing the Ketogenic Diet:

1. Educate Yourself

Before embarking on the ketogenic diet, it is crucial to invest time in comprehensive research and gain a thorough understanding of its basic underlying principles. Educating yourself about the ketogenic diet will allow you to make informed decisions and navigate the challenges that may arise during your keto journey.

You will also become more familiar with the fundamental concepts and guidelines that shape its implementation. This includes understanding macronutrient ratios, particularly the emphasis on low-carbohydrate intake, moderate protein consumption, and high-fat sources. Educating yourself about suitable food choices will enable you to make well-informed decisions when selecting the right ingredients for your keto meals and recipes.

Additionally, delving into meal planning strategies specific to the ketogenic diet will provide you with a roadmap to success. By considering factors such as portion sizes, nutrient balance, and variety, you will be able to optimize your nutritional intake while adhering to the basic ketogenic principles. Equipping yourself with meal planning knowledge will help you create well-balanced and enjoyable keto meals that align with your health and fitness goals.

Furthermore, learning about the potential challenges associated with the ketogenic diet will prepare you for any obstacles that may arise. This could include understanding the initial adjustment period known as the "keto flu," which can involve temporary symptoms, such as fatigue, headaches, or cravings. Being aware of these challenges and knowing how to mitigate their impact will lead to a smoother and more efficient transition into the ketogenic lifestyle.

2. Calculate Your Macronutrient Ratios

A key aspect of implementing the ketogenic diet is determining the optimal macronutrient ratios that align with your personal health goals and needs. These ratios are designed to induce and maintain a state of ketosis in the body, making it to rely predominantly on fat for fuel rather than carbohydrates.

In a standard ketogenic diet, the macronutrient distribution typically involves a high proportion of fat, a moderate intake of protein, and a minimal amount of carbohydrates. The recommended macronutrient ratios for a ketogenic diet commonly range around 70-75% of calories coming from fat, 20-25% from protein, and 5-10% from carbohydrates. However, it is important to note that these ranges may vary depending on individual factors, such as metabolic health, activity level, and specific dietary needs.

Calculating your macronutrient ratios involves determining the appropriate calorie intake from each macronutrient category. This can be achieved by multiplying your total daily calorie goal by the desired percentage contribution of each macronutrient. For example, if your daily calorie goal is 2000 calories, you would aim for approximately 1400-1500 calories from fat, 400-500 calories from protein, and 100-200 calories from carbohydrates.

As with any diet, these macronutrient ratios are not fixed and may require adjustment based on individual responses, goals, and metabolic factors. Some individuals may benefit from slightly higher or lower proportions of certain macronutrients.

3. Emphasize Healthy Fats

A crucial aspect of the ketogenic diet is prioritizing the consumption of healthy fats. Since the diet focuses on reducing carbohydrates, fats become the primary source of energy for the body. Incorporating a diverse range of healthy fat sources into your diet is essential for achieving the desired macronutrient balance and obtaining the necessary nutrients for overall health and well-being.

Healthy fats play a vital role in the ketogenic diet as they provide a concentrated source of energy and nutrients, and support various physiological functions within the body. Some examples of healthy fats suitable for the ketogenic diet include:

• **Olive Oil:** Rich in monounsaturated fats, olive oil is a staple in Mediterranean cuisine. It offers various benefits for heart health and contains antioxidants that combat inflammation.

• **Coconut Oil:** A great source of medium-chain triglycerides (MCTs), coconut oil is easily converted into ketones by the liver and serves as a readily available source of energy for the body. MCTs are known for their quick absorption, cognitive benefits, and anti-inflammatory effects.

• **Cocoa Butter:** Derived from cocoa beans, cocoa butter is a solid fat that provides a creamy texture to foods. It contains healthy saturated fats and antioxidants, which have beneficial effects on cardiovascular health.

• **Avocados:** Avocados are rich in monounsaturated fats and fiber, making them a valuable addition to the ketogenic diet. They also provide important vitamins, minerals, trace elements, and phytonutrients.

- **Nuts and Seeds:** Nuts and seeds are excellent sources of healthy fats, including omega-3 fatty acids, which have anti-inflammatory properties. Examples include almonds, walnuts, chia seeds, and flaxseeds.

Incorporating these healthy fat sources into your meals and snacks helps meet your caloric needs and provides a range of essential nutrients. Additionally, these fats contribute to satiety, helping you feel fuller for longer and supporting overall dietary adherence.

4. Moderate Protein Intake

Protein is an essential macronutrient that plays a crucial role in various physiological processes, including muscle growth, tissue repair, and hormone production. However, when following the ketogenic diet, it is important to moderate protein intake to ensure you stay in ketosis.

Excessive protein consumption can throw you out of ketosis due to a physiological process called gluconeogenesis. Gluconeogenesis occurs when the body, in the absence of sufficient carbohydrates, converts amino acids from protein into glucose to meet its energy needs. This can lead to an increase in blood glucose levels and inhibit the production of ketones, which are the primary fuel source in a ketogenic state.

To maintain an appropriate protein intake on the ketogenic diet, it is recommended to prioritize high-quality protein sources. These may include:

- **Quality Meats:** Opt for both lean and fatty cuts of meat, such as grass-fed beef, pasture-raised poultry, and pork. These meats provide essential amino acids and important micronutrients while being low in carbs.

- **Wild-Caught Fish:** Fatty fish like salmon, mackerel, and sardines are excellent sources of protein and omega-3 fatty acids. They contribute to overall health and provide anti-inflammatory benefits.

- **Plant-Based Protein Options:** For those following a vegetarian or vegan ketogenic diet, plant-based protein sources can be incorporated. Examples include tofu, tempeh, edamame, and certain nuts and seeds.

It is important to note that individual protein needs may vary based on factors such as activity level, age, sex, and overall health status.

5. Choose Low-Carb Vegetables

Choosing low-carb vegetables as the primary source of carbohydrates in the ketogenic diet is a key strategy to stay in ketosis while ensuring a nutrient-rich and balanced diet. Non-starchy vegetables offer numerous health benefits and are an excellent addition to a well-rounded ketogenic diet. Here are some reasons you should prioritize low-carb vegetables:

- **Fiber content:** Non-starchy vegetables are rich in dietary fiber, which plays a vital role in digestive health, satiety, and blood sugar control. Fiber helps regulate bowel movements, promotes the growth of beneficial gut bacteria, and contributes to feelings of fullness, aiding in weight management. Including fiber-rich vegetables in the ketogenic diet helps offset the low fiber intake often associated with low-carb eating plans.

- **Vitamins and minerals:** Non-starchy vegetables are packed with essential vitamins and minerals necessary for optimal health. Leafy greens like spinach, kale, and Swiss chard are abundant in vitamins A, C, and K, as well as folate and various minerals such as iron and magnesium. Broccoli and cauliflower are excellent sources of vitamin C, folate, and several minerals, including potassium. Zucchini and peppers provide vitamins A and C, along with other antioxidants. These nutrients support immune function, tissue repair, energy production, and numerous metabolic processes.

- **Phytonutrients and antioxidants:** Non-starchy vegetables contain a wide array of phytonutrients (such as lutein, carotenoids, and flavonoids) and antioxidants, which have been associated with numerous health benefits. These bioactive compounds have been shown to possess anti-inflammatory, anticancer, and cardiovascular protective properties. By including a diverse range of vegetables in the ketogenic diet, individuals can benefit from the unique phytonutrient profiles of different plant foods.

- **Low in calories and carbohydrates:** Non-starchy vegetables are generally low in calories and carbohydrates, making them suitable for maintaining ketosis and managing weight. They provide bulk and texture to meals without significantly impacting blood sugar levels. This allows individuals following the ketogenic diet to enjoy a variety of flavorful and satisfying foods while still adhering to their macronutrient goals.

When incorporating low-carb vegetables into the ketogenic diet, it's important to focus on non-starchy options. These include leafy greens, cruciferous vegetables (e.g., broccoli, cauliflower, Brussels sprouts), zucchini, peppers, cucumber, asparagus, mushrooms, and more. These vegetables typically have a low glycemic index and carbohydrate content, making them suitable for maintaining ketosis. To maximize the nutritional benefits of low-carb vegetables, it's advisable to consume them in their whole form rather than relying solely on processed or refined versions. Incorporating a variety of colors and types of vegetables ensures a diverse intake of nutrients and phytochemicals.

6. Stay Hydrated

Adequate hydration is crucial in any diet, but especially during the ketogenic diet. That's because when following keto, the body undergoes significant changes in its fluid and electrolyte balance. Firstly, the reduction in carbohydrate intake leads to a decrease in glycogen stores in the liver and muscles. Each gram of glycogen is stored with approximately 3-4 grams of water. As glycogen stores are depleted, water is released, resulting in increased urine output and potential water loss. This initial decrease in water weight is often observed during the first few days of starting a ketogenic diet.

Secondly, the ketogenic diet can have a diuretic effect due to the decrease in insulin levels. Insulin has an antidiuretic effect, meaning it promotes water reabsorption by the kidneys. As insulin levels decrease on the keto diet, the kidneys excrete more water along with electrolytes, such as sodium, potassium, and magnesium. This may lead to an increased risk of dehydration and electrolyte imbalances if adequate fluid and electrolyte replacement measures are not taken.

Furthermore, the body's metabolic shift into ketosis can increase water needs. When the body burns fat for fuel, ketones are produced as byproducts. Ketones are excreted through urine and breath, resulting in additional water loss. Therefore, during keto, maintaining proper hydration is essential to support the body's metabolic processes and prevent dehydration issues.

7. Monitor Ketone Levels

Monitoring ketone levels is a valuable tool for individuals following the ketogenic diet in order to assess their level of ketosis and track their progress. Ketones are byproducts of fat metabolism that serve as an alternative fuel source when carbohydrates are limited. Measuring ketone levels provides insight into the body's utilization of fat for energy.

There are several methods available for monitoring ketone levels, including:

- **Ketone Testing Strips:** Ketone testing strips, also known as ketone urine strips, are affordable and readily available for most. These strips detect the presence of ketones in urine by measuring the concentration of acetoacetate, one of the ketone bodies. While urine strips provide a convenient option, it's important to note that they may not be as accurate as other methods, especially for individuals who have been following the ketogenic diet for an extended period of time.

- **Blood Ketone Meters:** Blood ketone meters offer a more accurate and precise measurement of ketone levels. These devices require a small blood sample obtained through a finger prick. They measure the concentration of beta-hydroxybutyrate (BHB), the primary ketone body, in the blood. Blood ketone meters provide real-time results and are considered the gold standard for ketone level monitoring.

- **Breath Ketone Meters:** Breath ketone meters measure acetone, a ketone body, in the breath. These devices estimate ketone levels by detecting acetone on the breath and can provide a non-invasive alternative to blood or urine testing. However, breath ketone meters may have variations in accuracy and reliability.

When monitoring ketone levels, it's important to understand that the optimal range for ketosis can vary among individuals. Generally, a reading of 0.5 to 3.0 millimoles per liter (mmol/L) of blood ketones is considered indicative of nutritional ketosis. However, it's crucial to interpret ketone measurements in the context of individual goals, health status, and overall well-being.

The range of ketone levels can depend on factors such as the specific dietary approach, metabolic differences, and individual responses to the ketogenic diet. Some individuals may achieve and maintain ketosis at lower ketone levels, while others may require higher readings to experience the desired benefits.

Additionally, it's important to note that ketone levels alone do not guarantee the effectiveness or success of a ketogenic diet. Other factors, such as overall macronutrient composition, calorie intake, and individual health goals, should also be considered alongside ketone measurements.

Individual goals and health status should guide the interpretation of ketone levels. For example, those using the ketogenic diet for therapeutic purposes, such as managing epilepsy or certain medical conditions, may require more precise ketone monitoring and specific target ranges. On the other hand, individuals using the ketogenic diet for weight loss or general health and well-being may focus more on overall adherence and the benefits they experience rather than achieving specific ketone levels.

8. Meal Planning and Preparation

Meal planning and preparation are essential strategies for successfully implementing and sustaining the ketogenic diet. By planning your meals in advance, you can ensure that you have suitable options readily available and minimize the likelihood of making impulsive food choices that do not align with your dietary goals. Here are some key points to consider:

• **Set Aside Dedicated Time:** Allocate a specific time each week for meal planning and preparation. This can be a few hours on the weekend or any other day that works best for you. Having a designated time will help you stay organized and committed to your ketogenic eating plan.

• **Choose Keto-Friendly Recipes:** Look for recipes that are low in carbohydrates, high in healthy fats, and moderate in protein. There are numerous resources available, including cookbooks, online recipe websites, and mobile apps, that offer a wide range of delicious and satisfying ketogenic recipes. Experiment with different dishes to keep your meals varied, nutrient-dense, and enjoyable.

• **Create a Meal Plan:** Plan out your meals for the week, including breakfast, lunch, dinner, and snacks. Consider your macronutrient ratios and ensure that each meal is well-balanced and aligned with your specific dietary needs and goals. Incorporate a variety of nutrient-dense foods, including low-carb vegetables, healthy fats, and quality protein sources.

- **Make a Grocery List:** Based on your meal plan, create a comprehensive grocery list that includes all the ingredients you'll need for the week. This will help you stay organized while shopping and ensure that you have everything on hand when it's time to prepare your meals and recipes.

- **Batch Cooking and Portioning:** Consider batch cooking certain components of your meals, such as proteins, vegetables, or sauces, in advance. This can save you time and effort during the week. Once cooked, portion out the meals into individual containers, making it easy to grab a pre-portioned meal when you're on the go or busy.

- **Prep Snacks and Quick Meals:** Prepare keto-friendly snacks and quick meals that can be easily accessed when hunger strikes. This can include pre-cut vegetables, hard-boiled eggs, cheese slices, nuts, or homemade keto-friendly energy bars. Having these options readily available can help you avoid reaching out for carb-heavy snacks or convenience foods.

- **Utilize Storage Containers:** Invest in a variety of storage containers that are suitable for refrigerating or freezing your prepared meals. This will help maintain the freshness and quality of your food, and make it convenient to grab a meal when you need it.

By dedicating time to meal planning and preparation, you can ensure that your ketogenic diet is both sustainable and enjoyable. It allows you to stay in control of your food choices, maintain a well-balanced nutrient intake, and minimize the chances of deviating from your dietary goals.

9. Seek Professional Guidance: Before starting any new diet, especially one as specific as the ketogenic diet, it is crucial to seek professional guidance from a healthcare professional or a registered dietitian, particularly if you have underlying health conditions or concerns. Here's why it is important:

• **Personalized Advice:** Healthcare professionals and registered dietitians can provide personalized advice based on your individual health profile, medical history, and specific dietary needs. They can take into account factors such as any existing medical conditions, medications you may be taking, and your overall health goals.

• **Safety and Suitability:** Consulting with a professional ensures that the ketogenic diet is safe and suitable for you. They can assess any potential risks or contraindications, identify any necessary modifications to the diet, and provide recommendations that align with your health and longevity goals.

• **Optimal Nutrient Balance:** Professionals can help you achieve an optimal balance of nutrients while following the ketogenic diet. They can guide you in choosing the right sources of fats, proteins, and carbohydrates, ensuring that your diet remains nutritionally complete and promotes health and longevity.

• **Monitoring and Support:** Healthcare professionals and registered dietitians can monitor your progress and provide ongoing support throughout your ketogenic journey. They can help you navigate any challenges or setbacks, adjust your diet as needed, and provide guidance on managing any potential side effects or complications that may arise.

• Comprehensive Approach: Seeking professional guidance allows for a comprehensive approach to health and wellness. They can consider not only the dietary aspect but also other lifestyle factors that may impact your levels of well-being, such as physical activity, stress management, and sleep quality.

Summary

The ketogenic diet, with its emphasis on low-carbohydrate intake and high-fat consumption, has garnered attention for its potential benefits in various aspects of health and wellness. While keto offers promising results in terms of weight loss, improved insulin sensitivity, increased energy levels, and reduced inflammation, it is important to approach it with knowledge and awareness.

Implementing the ketogenic diet effectively starts with careful planning and understanding of its principles. Educating yourself about suitable food choices, meal planning, and potential challenges is crucial to ensure success and proper adherence. This knowledge will empower you to make informed decisions about your dietary choices and navigate potential obstacles that may arise along the way.

Choosing the right macronutrient ratios is essential in the ketogenic diet. Typically, this involves consuming approximately 70-75% of calories from fat, 20-25% from protein, and 5-10% from carbohydrates. These ratios may be adjusted based on individual needs, health goals, and tolerances.

Emphasizing healthy fats is a cornerstone of the ketogenic diet. Incorporating sources such as olive oil, coconut oil, cocoa butter, avocados, nuts, and seeds provides essential nutrients and helps meet caloric requirements. These healthy fats play a crucial role in fueling the body and supporting various physiological processes.

While protein is important for muscle growth and overall health, excessive protein consumption can hinder ketosis due to gluconeogenesis. The process of gluconeogenesis, where protein is converted into glucose for energy, can disrupt ketosis. Opting for moderate protein intake from quality sources such as lean and fatty cuts of meat, pasture-raised poultry, wild-caught fish, and plant-based options helps strike a balance between nutritional needs and staying in ketosis.

Monitoring ketone levels is a valuable tool to track progress and ensure that the body is actually in a state of ketosis. Ketone testing strips or blood ketone meters can provide insight into the body's metabolic state and help individuals make necessary adjustments to their diet and lifestyle.

Meal planning and preparation are powerful tools for success on the ketogenic diet. Planning meals in advance ensures suitable options are readily available, minimizing the likelihood of impulsive food choices. Preparing meals and snacks ahead of time promotes adherence to the diet and helps individuals stay on track.

Additionally, seeking professional guidance is oftentimes recommended, especially for individuals with underlying health conditions or concerns. Consulting with a healthcare professional or registered dietitian experienced in the ketogenic diet allows for personalized guidance, taking into account individual health profiles, medical history, and specific dietary needs. These professionals can provide expert advice, monitor progress, and ensure that the ketogenic diet is safe and suitable for each person.

Overall, the ketogenic diet offers a unique approach to nutrition with potential benefits in various areas of health and wellness. However, as with any diet, it is important to approach it with knowledge, awareness, and individual considerations. By understanding its principles, making informed choices, monitoring progress, and seeking professional guidance when necessary, you can implement the ketogenic diet safely and effectively.

Similarities and Differences Between the Carnivore and Ketogenic Diets

In this section, we will explore the similarities and differences between the carnivore and ketogenic diets, shedding light on their principles, food choices, potential benefits, and drawbacks. By examining these aspects, we can gain a comprehensive understanding of how these dietary approaches align and diverge.

Similarities

- **Carbohydrate Restriction:** One of the primary similarities between keto and carnivore is their emphasis on reducing carbohydrate intake. Both diets restrict the consumption of high-carb foods, such as grains, sugary treats, and starchy vegetables. By minimizing carbohydrate intake, both diets aim to promote a metabolic state known as ketosis, where the body primarily utilizes fat for energy instead of carbohydrates.

- **Focus on Healthy Fats:** Both diets emphasize the inclusion of healthy fats as a significant part of their macronutrient composition. While the carnivore diet primarily focuses on animal-based fats, such as those found in meat, fish, eggs, dairy products, and rendered animal fats, the ketogenic diet incorporates a wider variety of fat sources, including avocados, nuts, seeds, and oils. The consumption of healthy fats helps provide satiety, supports hormone production, and aids in the absorption of fat-soluble vitamins.

• **Potential Weight Loss:** Both carnivore and keto have been associated with weight loss benefits. By reducing carbohydrate intake and increasing fat consumption, these diets can promote satiety, stabilize blood sugar levels, and enhance fat burning. Additionally, the removal of processed foods and refined sugars in both diets positively contributes to weight loss and improved body composition.

Differences

• **Food Choices:** The most significant difference between the carnivore and ketogenic diets lies in their food choices. The carnivore diet revolves around animal-based foods and primarily consists of meat, fish, eggs, and dairy. It eliminates all plant-based foods, like fruits, vegetables, nuts, seeds, legumes, and grains. On the other hand, the ketogenic diet includes a more diverse range of food options, allowing for low-carb vegetables, nuts, seeds, and certain fruits (i.e. berries, lemons) in limited quantities.

• **Protein Intake:** While both diets advocate for a high fat intake, their protein recommendations differ. The carnivore diet encourages higher protein consumption, as it primarily relies on animal products as the main source of nutrition. In contrast, the ketogenic diet emphasizes moderate protein intake, as excess protein can potentially be converted to glucose through the process of gluconeogenesis, which can hinder ketosis.

- **Philosophical Approach:** Beyond their dietary composition, the carnivore and ketogenic diets have different underlying philosophies. The carnivore diet, also considered an ancestral diet, is rooted in the concept of mimicking the dietary patterns of early humans who subsisted mainly on animal products. It aims to eliminate potential allergens, immune system irritants, antinutrients, and processed foods. The ketogenic diet, on the other hand, was initially developed as an alternative therapeutic approach to manage epilepsy and later gained popularity as a weight loss and health optimization strategy.

- **Long-Term Sustainability:** The long-term sustainability of the carnivore and ketogenic diets is an area of disagreement. While both diets have shown short-term benefits, their long-term effects on overall health and nutritional adequacy are not fully understood. The elimination of entire food groups in the carnivore diet and the strict macronutrient ratios in the ketogenic diet may pose challenges in terms of nutritional diversity, nutrient adequacy, and adherence over extended periods.

Summary

The carnivore and ketogenic diets share certain similarities and have distinct differences that make them unique approaches to nutrition and health. Both diets restrict carbohydrate intake, emphasize the consumption of healthy fats, and have the potential for weight loss, improved metabolic health, and body recomposition. However, they differ in terms of food choices, protein intake, philosophical approach, and long-term sustainability.

The carnivore diet focuses exclusively on animal-based products, eliminating plant-based foods completely from the diet. It is often considered an ancestral approach to eating, attempting to mimic the dietary patterns of early humans. The carnivore diet promotes higher protein consumption than keto and aims to eliminate potential allergens, immune system irritants, and anti-nutrients. While it may offer benefits, such as reduced inflammation, weight loss, enhanced endocrine health, and better focus, its long-term sustainability is an open topic of debate.

On the other hand, the ketogenic diet allows for a wider range of food choices, including low-carb vegetables, nuts, seeds, and limited amounts of fruits. It originated as a therapeutic diet for epilepsy and has gained popularity as a weight loss and health optimization strategy. The ketogenic diet emphasizes moderate protein intake to prevent excess glucose production through gluconeogenesis and to maintain ketosis. It provides more flexibility in terms of food choices but adheres to strict and specific macronutrient ratios, which make its long-term sustainability a challenge for certain individuals.

When considering these diets, it is crucial to assess their potential benefits and drawbacks in the context of your own specific health goals, preferences, needs, and lifestyle. Both diets have shown promising short-term benefits, but more long-term research is needed to accurately assess their impact on overall health and longevity.

Effects on Metabolic Health and Weight Loss: Which One is Superior?

Both carnivore and keto have gained significant attention in recent years for their potential benefits on metabolic health, weight loss, and body composition. These two dietary approaches share certain similarities, such as carbohydrate restriction and emphasis on healthy fat consumption, but also exhibit distinct differences in terms of food choices and overall macronutrient composition.

In this section, we will compare the effects of these two diets on metabolic health markers and weight loss outcomes, shedding light on their potential benefits and considerations for individuals seeking to optimize their health and fitness through them.

Metabolic Health

Both the ketogenic and carnivore diets have shown potential in improving various markers of metabolic health. These two dietary approaches offer notable benefits in regulating blood sugar levels and enhancing insulin sensitivity, which are critical aspects of metabolic health. By limiting carbohydrate intake, both diets compel the body to rely on alternative fuel sources like fats and ketones, resulting in improved blood glucose control and reduced insulin resistance.

Research studies have consistently demonstrated the effectiveness of both diets in lowering fasting blood glucose and hemoglobin A1c levels, particularly in individuals with type II diabetes or insulin resistance. The carbohydrate restriction and metabolic adaptation induced by these diets contribute to better glycemic control, making them valuable tools for managing blood sugar levels.

Moreover, both the ketogenic and carnivore diets have displayed favorable effects on lipid profiles. These dietary approaches typically emphasize the consumption of healthy fats, such as monounsaturated fats and omega-3 fatty acids, while restricting processed carbohydrates and trans fats. This dietary pattern has been associated with increased levels of high-density lipoprotein (HDL) cholesterol, often referred to as the "good" cholesterol, and reduced levels of triglycerides, a type of fat linked to an increased risk of heart disease.

The strategic inclusion of healthy fats and the elimination of refined carbohydrates and trans fats contribute to the overall improvement in lipid profiles observed in individuals following these diets. The reduction in triglyceride levels and the increase in HDL cholesterol are indicative of a more favorable lipid status and a lower risk of cardiovascular disease.

Weight Loss

Both carnivore and keto have gained recognition as effective dietary strategies for weight loss. The key mechanism behind their weight loss benefits lies in the reduction of carbohydrate intake, which leads to decreased insulin levels and promotes the utilization of stored body fat for energy.

The ketogenic diet has been extensively studied for its weight loss benefits. By inducing a state of nutritional ketosis, where the body primarily relies on fat for fuel, individuals may experience reduced appetite, increased satiety, and enhanced fat metabolism. This can result in significant weight loss, particularly in the initial stages of the diet. However, it is important to note that adhering to the strict macronutrient ratios of the ketogenic diet and managing potential side effects, such as the notorious "keto flu," can present certain challenges for some individuals.

On the other hand, the weight loss effects of the carnivore diet have been less extensively studied. Due to its emphasis on protein consumption, which is highly satiating and thermogenic (a.k.a. fat-burning), individuals following the carnivore diet may experience reduced hunger and improved portion control, ultimately leading to weight loss. However, more long-term studies are needed to fully assess the sustainability and potential drawbacks of this way of eating.

Considerations and Potential Drawbacks

While the carnivore and ketogenic diets offer several benefits for metabolic health and weight loss, it is important to consider potential drawbacks and individual considerations.

Firstly, both diets can pose certain challenges in terms of nutrient adequacy and potential deficiencies. The carnivore diet, which eliminates all plant-based foods, may be lacking in certain vitamins, minerals, trace elements, fiber, and phytonutrients commonly found in fruits, vegetables, nuts, seeds, and whole grains. On the other hand, the ketogenic diet may require careful planning to ensure sufficient intake of essential nutrients, such as vitamins, minerals, trace elements, and fiber, from low-carb, plant-based sources.

Additionally, the sustainability of these two diets is a key consideration. The highly restrictive nature of the carnivore diet and the strict macronutrient ratios of the ketogenic diet can make long-term adherence challenging for a lot of people. Social and cultural factors, personal food preferences, and practicality in daily life should also be taken into account when considering these two diets.

Furthermore, it is important to note that individual responses to the carnivore and ketogenic diets may vary. While some individuals may experience significant improvements in metabolic health markers and weight loss, others may not respond as favorably or may even experience adverse effects. Factors such as genetics, underlying health conditions, and overall lifestyle should all be considered when determining the suitability of these diets for an individual.

Moreover, the long-term effects of the carnivore and ketogenic diets on overall health and chronic disease prevention are still largely unknown. While short-term studies have shown promising results, there is a need for more extensive research to assess the potential risks and drawbacks over extended periods.

Summary

The carnivore and ketogenic diets share certain similarities in terms of carbohydrate restriction and emphasis on fat consumption, making them potentially effective dietary approaches for metabolic health improvement and weight loss. Both diets have demonstrated favorable effects on blood sugar control, insulin sensitivity, and lipid profiles. However, their long-term effects and sustainability require further investigation.

Individual considerations, such as nutrient adequacy, long-term adherence, and potential drawbacks, should all be taken into account when deciding whether to adopt one of these two diets. Consulting with a healthcare professional or registered dietitian experienced in one or both of these dietary approaches can provide personalized guidance and support in choosing the most appropriate option based on individual health goals, needs, preferences, and lifestyle factors.

Alternating Between the Ketogenic and Carnivore Diets

Alternating between the ketogenic and carnivore diets can be a practical solution for individuals finding long-term adherence to a strict carnivore diet challenging or unsustainable. While the carnivore diet can be a highly effective dietary approach in terms of health and weight loss, it may become overly restrictive during social events or special occasions where a wider variety of foods are enjoyed by others. The desire to partake in these culinary and social experiences can be a significant barrier to long-term adherence.

One potential strategy to manage issues like this is to incorporate periodic cycles of carnivore nutrition with phases of the ketogenic diet. By adopting this alternating approach, individuals may get to experience the amazing benefits of both diets while allowing for greater flexibility in terms of food choices during certain periods. For instance, a person may choose to follow a strict, nose-to-tail carnivore diet for a duration of 6 to 10 weeks, two or three times a year, and then transition to a structured, well-balanced, and clean ketogenic diet for the subsequent period.

During the carnivore phase, the focus should remain on consuming animal-based foods only, emphasizing nutrient-dense options, such as fatty cuts of grass-fed meat, organ meats, eggs, raw dairy, and bone broth. This phase provides the opportunity to reap the amazing benefits of the carnivore diet, including improved metabolic health, reduced inflammation, improved hormone status, and weight loss. The absence of plant-based foods during this period eliminates most potential allergens or irritants that are typically present in people's diets.

After the carnivore phase, transitioning to a ketogenic phase allows for the reintroduction of a broader range of food options while still maintaining the benefits of carbohydrate restriction. This cyclic nature of alternating between carnivore and keto offers several advantages. Firstly, it provides a psychological reprieve by allowing dieters to enjoy a wider variety of foods during social gatherings or special events without feeling restricted. This can contribute to better adherence and overall satisfaction with the dietary regimen, which is extremely important. Additionally, cycling between the two diets exposes the body to different nutrient profiles and can potentially enhance nutrient diversity and overall nutritional status.

Furthermore, the periodic transition between the carnivore and ketogenic diets helps prevent adaptation and plateauing. As you may already know, the body's metabolic response can gradually adjust to a specific dietary pattern over time, potentially leading to a reduction in the effectiveness of the diet. By alternating between the carnivore and ketogenic diets, individuals can achieve variation and metabolic flexibility, which improves their body's response to dietary interventions.

Summary

Alternating between the ketogenic and carnivore diets may provide a more balanced and effective approach to optimizing health, as this approach combines the benefits of both dietary strategies. By incorporating cycles of the carnivore diet, individuals can experience the amazing metabolic advantages and weight loss benefits this diet has to offer, while also allowing for more flexibility and enjoyment during social occasions. Transitioning to a ketogenic diet during other periods maintains the advantages of carbohydrate restriction and can support long-term metabolic health and weight loss.

How To Transition From Keto To Carnivore

Transitioning from a ketogenic diet that also includes some plants to a strict carnivore diet that excludes them altogether can be approached simply and gradually. Below are some steps to consider when making this transition:

1. Analyze Your Food Journal: Start by keeping a detailed food journal to track your calorie and macronutrient intake. Highlight all animal-based foods in your journal to determine what percentage of your current diet comes from animals vs. plants. This will provide you with a baseline understanding of your current eating patterns.

2. Calculate Your Calorie Intake from Plants: Once you have a clear picture of your current food intake, determine how many calories you obtain from plant foods. This will help you determine what portion of your diet needs to be replaced with animal products when transitioning to a carnivore diet. If you are at a healthy weight, aim to maintain the same number of calories. If weight loss is the goal, consider reducing your calorie intake slightly.

3. Gradually Replace Greens with Meat: Over a period of 7-10 days, gradually remove plant-based items from your diet and increase your consumption of meat. This gradual transition will allow your body to adapt better and will minimize the risk of feeling drained, depleted, or weak during the process. It will also allow you to maintain your exercise routine without significant disruptions or drops in performance.

4. Diversify the Meats You Eat: To make your carnivore diet more enjoyable and nutritionally diverse, incorporate a variety of meats into your meals. Experiment with different types of meat, such as beef, lamb, bison, buffalo, pork, chicken, fatty fish, and organ meats (offal). Food variety not only improves compliance with the diet, but also provides a broader range of essential nutrients.

5. Monitor Your Ketone Levels: As you reduce your carbohydrate intake and increase your meat consumption, you may notice an increase in your ketone levels. Ketones can be measured using special devices and test strips that analyze ketone levels in the urine, blood, and breath. Higher ketone levels are generally considered a positive indicator of moving in the right direction. Monitoring your ketone levels throughout the day, noting the measurements, and tracking your mood will provide motivation and insight into how your body responds to the dietary modifications.

6. Everyone is Different: Remember that each individual's experience may vary, and it is essential to listen to your own body and make adjustments accordingly. Gradual transitions and regular monitoring help optimize the transition process from a ketogenic diet to a carnivore diet, while maintaining optimum levels of health, well-being, and performance.

Keto vs. Carnivore: Which One Is Better?

The debate between the ketogenic and carnivore diets often revolves around which one is superior. It is important to note here that these diets are not necessarily mutually exclusive or in direct competition with each other. In fact, they can be seen as complementary approaches to achieving specific health or body composition goals. For those new to dietary interventions, starting with the ketogenic diet first and then gradually transitioning into a carnivore diet with regular cycling between the two can be a simple, smooth, and effective approach.

The ketogenic diet involves significantly reducing your carbohydrate intake and increasing fat consumption to induce a state of ketosis, where your body primarily relies on fat for fuel. This metabolic shift can have various health benefits, including weight loss, increased insulin sensitivity, and improved mental clarity. The emphasis on consuming high-quality fats, moderate protein, and low carbohydrates distinguishes the keto diet from a plain low-carb diet.

On the other hand, the carnivore diet takes the concept of carbohydrate restriction to a whole new level, focusing exclusively on animal-based products while eliminating plants. This diet emphasizes consuming meat, including muscle meat, organ meats, and animal fats, while avoiding carbohydrates, fiber, and plant-based foods and byproducts. Advocates of the carnivore diet claim benefits such as reduced inflammation, improved mental well-being, better gut health, enhanced energy levels, increased libido, and better recovery from exercise.

While both diets share the common feature of carbohydrate restriction, they differ in terms of food choices and overall macronutrient composition. The keto diet allows for a broader range of food options, including high-fat plant-based foods, like avocados, nuts, and seeds, whereas the carnivore diet strictly limits food choices to animal-based sources.

For individuals who find it challenging to commit to the strict guidelines of either the keto or carnivore diet, reducing their carbohydrate intake alone may still yield some results. A low-carb diet, followed long enough, can help stabilize blood sugar levels, promote weight loss, and improve insulin sensitivity and overall metabolic health. It can also serve as a stepping stone towards other more specialized dietary interventions (e.g. carnivore or keto).

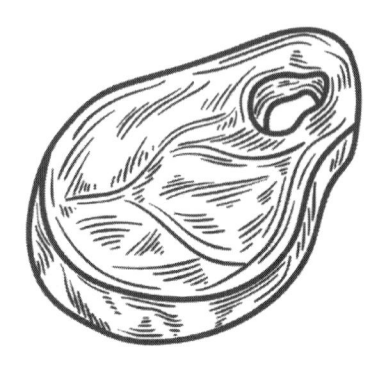

CHAPTER 4: 40+ CARNIVORE DIET FAQS

As the carnivore diet continues to gain popularity, it is natural for individuals to have questions and concerns regarding its safety, implementation, sustainability, and potential side effects. In this section, we have compiled a list of frequently asked questions about the carnivore diet and provided evidence-based information to help you make well-informed decisions.

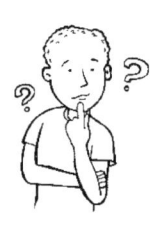

1. Is the Carnivore Diet Nutritionally Balanced?

The carnivore diet, characterized by the exclusion of plant-based foods and the emphasis on animal-based foods, can be nutritionally balanced if certain considerations are taken into account. Animal-based foods, such as meat, poultry, fish, eggs, and dairy, are rich sources of quality protein, essential fatty acids, vitamins, minerals, trace elements, and other compounds. These nutrients are crucial for various physiologic and metabolic processes within the body.

Protein is a key component of the carnivore diet, as animal-based proteins are considered complete proteins, containing all the essential amino acids necessary for bodily functions, including muscle repair, growth, and various metabolic processes. Adequate protein intake is important for maintaining lean body mass and supporting overall health.

Healthy fats, found abundantly in animal sources like fatty cuts of meat and certain types of fatty fish, are essential for hormone production, nutrient absorption, inflammation regulation, and cellular function. These fats provide a concentrated source of energy and contribute to satiety, making them an important component of any healthy diet.

Animal-based foods also provide essential vitamins, minerals, and trace elements, including vitamin B12, iron, zinc, and selenium. Vitamin B12, primarily found in animal products, is essential for nerve function and the production of red blood cells. Iron is important for oxygen transport and energy production, while zinc and selenium play crucial roles in immune function, endocrine health, and antioxidant defence.

However, careful attention should be given to certain nutrients that may be lacking or less abundant in the carnivore diet due to the complete exclusion of plant-based foods. Fiber, primarily found in fruits, vegetables, nuts, seeds, legumes, and whole grains, is important for digestive health, satiety, and maintaining a diverse gut microbiota. Lack of fiber in the diet can lead to changes in bowel movements and potentially affect gut health.

Additionally, some vitamins, such as vitamin C, are predominantly found in plant-based foods. Vitamin C is a potent antioxidant and plays a critical role in collagen synthesis, immune function, and wound healing. While it is true that some animal-based foods, like liver and certain fish, contain small amounts of vitamin C, these levels are a lot lower than plant-based sources.

Phytochemicals, including various antioxidants and bioactive compounds (i.e. carotenoids, polyphenols, etc), are abundant in fruits, vegetables, and other plant-based foods. These compounds have been associated with numerous health benefits, including reducing the risk of chronic diseases. The absence of plants in the carnivore diet may limit the intake of these beneficial compounds.

To maintain nutritional balance in the carnivore diet, adjustments, and supplementation may be necessary. Incorporating organ meats, which are extremely nutrient-dense, can provide a wider array of vitamins, minerals, and trace elements. Supplementation with certain nutrients like vitamin C or fiber sources may also be considered to address potential deficiencies and problems.

Regular monitoring of nutrient status through blood tests and consultations with healthcare professionals or registered dietitians (ideally experienced in the carnivore diet) can help ensure that your nutritional needs are being met. Individual variations in nutrient requirements, goals, and health conditions should also be taken into account when tailoring the carnivore diet for optimal health and wellness outcomes.

2. Can the Carnivore Diet Lead to Nutrient Deficiencies?

The carnivore diet can lead to certain nutrient deficiencies if not carefully planned and monitored. Although animal-based foods provide an abundance of essential nutrients, the complete absence of plant-based foods may result in inadequate intake of certain dietary components.

One potential concern on the carnivore diet is the lack of dietary fiber. Fiber, found abundantly in fruits, vegetables, nuts, seeds, legumes, and whole grains, plays a crucial role in promoting regular bowel movements, maintaining gut health, and supporting a diverse gut microbiota. Without adequate fiber intake, individuals on the carnivore diet may experience changes in bowel habits and an increased risk of constipation.

In terms of vitamins, some may be less abundant or completely absent in the carnivore diet. Vitamin C, for example, is predominantly found in fruits and vegetables and is essential for various biological functions in the body, including collagen synthesis, immune function, and antioxidant defence. While it is true that certain animal-based foods contain small amounts of vitamin C, they do not provide enough to meet daily requirements. Consequently, individuals following the carnivore diet may need to consider vitamin C supplementation or explore alternative sources, such as certain organ meats.

Mineral deficiencies may also be a concern, especially if the carnivore diet lacks variety. While animal-based foods are generally rich in minerals like iron, zinc, and selenium, the absence of plant-based foods may limit the intake of certain minerals and trace elements found predominantly in those sources. For instance, plant-based foods can be important sources of magnesium and potassium. Monitoring mineral levels through blood tests and considering targeted supplementation, if necessary, can help mitigate potential deficiencies.

Antioxidants, such as various phytochemicals found in fruits, vegetables, and other plant-based foods, are important for reducing oxidative stress and combating inflammation in the body. The exclusion of these foods from the carnivore diet may result in reduced antioxidant intake.

However, it is worth noting that certain animal-based foods, such as liver, contain antioxidants like vitamin A, vitamin E, and selenium, which contribute to the overall antioxidant potency of the diet.

To prevent nutrient deficiencies in the carnivore diet, careful attention should be given to nutrient intake (e.g. ensure a diverse selection of animal-based foods) and considering targeted supplementation when necessary. Regular blood tests, including comprehensive nutrient panels, can help assess nutrient status and identify any deficiencies. Working with a healthcare professional or registered dietitian who has experience with the carnivore diet can provide valuable guidance in ensuring nutritional adequacy while on the diet.

It is important to keep in mind that individual nutrient needs may vary based on factors such as age, sex, physical activity level, and health status. Therefore, a personalized approach is recommended when addressing nutrient deficiencies and optimizing nutrient intake on the carnivore diet.

3. What is the Impact of the Carnivore Diet on Gut Health?

The impact of the carnivore diet on gut health is a complex and evolving topic that warrants further investigation. While some individuals may experience improvements in digestive symptoms, such as reduced bloating and gas, upon adopting the carnivore diet, the long-term effects on gut health and microbiota diversity are not yet fully understood.

The gut microbiota, consisting of trillions of microorganisms that reside in the gastrointestinal tract, plays a critical role in various aspects of human health and physiology, including digestion, immune function, and metabolism. A diverse and balanced gut microbiota is generally associated with better health outcomes.

One aspect of the carnivore diet that may influence gut health is the elimination of plant-based foods. Plants contain various types of dietary fibers that serve as prebiotics, which act as food for beneficial gut bacteria. These prebiotics help nourish and support the growth of beneficial bacteria in the gut, contributing to a diverse and healthy gut microbiome.

The exclusion of plant-based foods in the carnivore diet means that individuals may have limited intake of these prebiotic fibers, which can potentially impact the composition and diversity of the gut microbiota. Research suggests that a reduction in dietary fiber intake can lead to a decrease in the presence of fiber-degrading bacteria, potentially compromising gut health.

To support gut health while following the carnivore diet, it is important to consider strategies to maintain a healthy gut microbiome. Including fermented foods, such as goat's milk products (i.e. yogurt or kefir), in the diet can provide beneficial probiotic bacteria that support gut health. Fermented foods contain live microorganisms that can colonize the gut and contribute to a better diversity of gut bacteria.

Additionally, considering high-quality probiotic supplements may be beneficial for supporting a healthier gut microbiome. Probiotics are live microorganisms that, when administered in adequate amounts, confer health benefits to the host. They can help restore and maintain a balanced gut microbiota, especially when the diet lacks certain fiber-rich plant foods.

It is worth noting that individual responses to dietary changes can vary, including the impact on gut health. Some individuals may experience improvements in digestive symptoms when following the carnivore diet, while others may not observe significant changes or even experience adverse effects. Monitoring gut health markers, such as changes in bowel movements (i.e. frequency, stool consistency, etc), can provide valuable insights into individual responses and inform any necessary adjustments to the diet.

Overall, the impact of the carnivore diet on gut health is a complex and multifaceted topic that requires further scientific investigation. Prioritizing gut health by incorporating well-sourced fermented dairy products (i.e. yogurt or kefir made from organic, grass-fed milk) and considering high-quality probiotic supplements, if necessary, can be valuable strategies to support a healthy gut microbiome while following the carnivore diet.

4. How Does the Carnivore Diet Affect Cholesterol Levels?

The effects of the carnivore diet on cholesterol levels are a subject of ongoing research and debate. While individual responses may vary, several studies have suggested that adopting the carnivore diet may lead to changes in cholesterol profiles, including increased levels of total cholesterol, LDL (often referred to as "bad" cholesterol), and HDL (considered "good" cholesterol). However, it is crucial to approach the interpretation of these changes and their implications for cardiovascular health with careful consideration.

Total cholesterol represents the overall amount of cholesterol in the blood, comprising both LDL and HDL cholesterol. Elevated levels of LDL cholesterol have been associated with an increased risk of cardiovascular disease, while HDL cholesterol plays a role in transporting cholesterol away from tissues.

Research exploring the impact of the carnivore diet on cholesterol levels has produced mixed results. Some individuals may experience increases in both LDL and HDL cholesterol, while others may witness minimal changes or even reductions. The response to the diet may depend on various factors, including genetic predisposition, baseline cholesterol levels, and overall metabolic health.

However, it is essential to recognize that changes in cholesterol levels alone do not provide a comprehensive assessment of cardiovascular health. Factors such as inflammation, blood pressure, and blood glucose levels also contribute significantly to assessing overall cardiovascular risk. Thus, considering these factors alongside cholesterol levels is crucial when evaluating cardiovascular health.

Regular monitoring of cholesterol levels is advisable for individuals adhering to the carnivore diet, particularly for those with pre-existing cardiovascular risk factors. This facilitates ongoing assessment and enables informed decision-making regarding dietary modifications or the need for additional interventions.

Consulting with healthcare professionals, including registered dietitians or physicians specializing in lipid management, can provide valuable guidance in understanding individual risk factors and interpreting changes in cholesterol levels within the context of the carnivore diet. These professionals can help develop personalized dietary strategies and offer recommendations to mitigate potential risks associated with cholesterol level changes.

It is important to acknowledge that the impact of the carnivore diet on cardiovascular health is still an area of active research, and further studies are needed to fully understand its long-term implications. Individual responses to dietary interventions can vary significantly, and what may be suitable for one person may not be appropriate for another. Thus, taking a personalized approach and maintaining ongoing monitoring are key when considering the effects of the carnivore diet on cholesterol levels and overall cardiovascular health.

5. Is the Carnivore Diet Sustainable Long Term?

The long-term sustainability of the carnivore diet requires careful consideration and attention to potential impacts on overall health and well-being. While some individuals may choose to adhere to the carnivore diet for extended periods, it is essential to assess the potential risks and benefits associated with this dietary approach.

A primary concern surrounding the long-term sustainability of the carnivore diet is the risk of nutrient deficiencies. By excluding plant-based foods, individuals following the carnivore diet may be at a higher likelihood of inadequate intake of certain nutrients, including fiber, vitamins (such as vitamin C), minerals, trace elements, and phytochemicals found in fruits, vegetables, nuts, seeds, and whole grains. To mitigate this risk, it is crucial to pay close attention to nutrient intake and consider incorporating a wide range of nutrient-dense animal foods into the diet. Additionally, targeted supplementation may be necessary to address any potential nutrient gaps.

Emphasizing nutrient-dense organ meats can be beneficial in addressing some of the potential nutrient deficiencies associated with the carnivore diet. Organ meats, such as liver and heart, are particularly rich in essential vitamins and minerals, including iron, vitamin A, vitamin B12, and folate. Incorporating a variety of animal-based foods, such as beef, poultry, fish, eggs, and dairy, can also contribute to a more diverse nutrient profile and help support long-term nutritional adequacy.

Regular monitoring of health markers, including blood tests and other relevant assessments, is crucial in evaluating the impact of the carnivore diet on overall health. These evaluations can help identify any imbalances or deficiencies that may arise and allow for timely interventions to maintain optimal health and prevent any negative health consequences.

Collaborating with healthcare professionals or registered dietitians who have experience with the carnivore diet can provide valuable guidance and support for long-term sustainability. They can help develop personalized strategies to ensure nutrient adequacy, monitor health markers, and address any potential concerns that may arise.

It is important to note that the long-term effects of the carnivore diet on various health outcomes are still not fully understood. Individual responses to the diet can vary, and what may work for one person may not work for another. Applying an individualized approach to nutrition and considering personal health goals, medical history, and other factors are crucial when evaluating the long-term sustainability of the carnivore diet or any diet.

6. What Are the Potential Risks Associated With the Carnivore Diet?

The carnivore diet, like any dietary approach, comes with potential risks and considerations that individuals should be aware of. It is important to evaluate these risks and take appropriate measures to mitigate them. Here are some of the potential risks associated with the carnivore diet:

1. Nutrient Deficiencies: The elimination of plant-based foods in the carnivore diet can lead to potential nutrient deficiencies. Fiber, found in fruits, vegetables, nuts, seeds, legumes, and whole grains, plays a crucial role in digestive health and the prevention of certain diseases. Furthermore, plant-based foods are rich sources of various vitamins, minerals, trace elements, and phytonutrients (i.e. carotenoids, ellagic acid, flavonoids, resveratrol, etc) that are important for overall health. Careful planning, monitoring nutrient intake, and potentially incorporating targeted supplementation can help prevent nutrient deficiencies in the carnivore diet.

2. Limited Antioxidant Intake: Fruits and vegetables are abundant sources of antioxidants, which help protect the body against oxidative stress and inflammation. By eliminating or greatly reducing these foods, individuals on the carnivore diet may have limited antioxidant intake. Oxidative stress and chronic inflammation are associated with the development of various diseases. Therefore, alternative strategies should be considered to ensure adequate antioxidant intake on the carnivore diet, such as consuming antioxidant-rich animal foods, like organ meats and certain types of fish (i.e. salmon) and seafood.

3. Impact on Cardiovascular Health: The high intake of saturated fats and cholesterol from animal sources may raise some concerns about cardiovascular health. Saturated fats have been associated with an increased risk of heart disease in some studies. However, it is important to note that the relationship between saturated fats and cardiovascular health is quite complex and still under scientific investigation. It is advisable to monitor lipid profiles, including cholesterol levels, and consult with healthcare professionals to assess individual risk factors and make informed dietary decisions.

4. Potential Adverse Effects on Gut Health: The complete exclusion of plant-based foods may impact gut health by reducing the diversity of gut microbiota. A diverse and balanced gut microbiome is important for various health aspects, including digestion, immune function, and mental well-being. To support gut health, individuals following the carnivore diet should consider incorporating fermented animal-based foods, such as goat's milk yogurt or kefir, and possibly probiotic supplementation.

5. Social and Practical Challenges: Following the carnivore diet may present certain social and practical challenges. For example, it may be difficult to find suitable food options when dining out or attending social events, as most establishments and gatherings typically offer a variety of foods that may not align with the restrictions of the carnivore diet. Additionally, adhering to a hyper-restrictive eating pattern can be challenging for a lot of people, potentially affecting their overall satisfaction and adherence to the diet.

To mitigate these risks, it is crucial to assess individual health factors, monitor biomarkers (such as blood lipid levels), and consult with healthcare professionals, including registered dietitians, who are experienced in low-carb eating and can provide personalized guidance and support. They can help develop personalized strategies to ensure nutrient adequacy, address potential risks, and monitor overall health status while on the carnivore diet.

7. Can the Carnivore Diet Be Followed by Athletes or Individuals With High Energy Demands?

The carnivore diet can be followed by athletes or individuals with high energy demands, but it requires careful consideration and adjustments to ensure that energy intake, nutrient balance, and recovery are adequately addressed. Here are some important key factors to consider when adapting the carnivore diet for athletes or those with high energy needs:

• **Energy Intake:** Athletes or individuals with high energy demands typically require more calories to fuel their physical activity and support optimal performance. Since the carnivore diet is often low in carbohydrates, which are a primary source of energy for the body, it becomes important to ensure sufficient energy intake from other macronutrients. This may involve increasing the portion sizes of protein, but especially fat sources, or incorporating energy-dense animal-based foods to meet energy requirements, such as fatty cuts of meat and full-fat dairy products (i.e. butter, cream, cheese, etc).

• **Protein Intake:** Protein is essential for muscle repair, recovery, and growth. Athletes or individuals with high energy demands typically require a higher protein intake to support their training needs. Animal-based proteins, such as meat, poultry, fish, and eggs, are complete proteins that provide all the essential amino acids necessary for muscle protein synthesis (MPS), which is the process by which the body builds new muscle proteins or repairs damaged muscle fibers. MPS is a key mechanism involved in muscle growth, adaptation, and recovery from exercise. Thus, adequate protein intake, spread throughout the day, should be prioritized to support muscle recovery, growth, and training adaptation.

- **Fat Intake:** Fat is an important source of energy and should be increased to compensate for the reduced carbohydrate intake in the carnivore diet. Including healthy sources of fats, such as fatty cuts of meat, fatty fish, whole eggs, full-fat dairy, and rendered animal fats (i.e. tallow, lard, duck fat), can help meet energy needs. It is important to choose quality fats that provide essential fatty acids and fat-soluble vitamins (A, D, E, K).

- **Nutrient Timing:** Strategic timing of meals and nutrient intake can help optimize athletic performance and recovery. Pre- and post-workout nutrition should be carefully considered to provide the necessary macronutrients and energy to support muscle repair and growth. Including a source of high-quality protein before and after workouts, along with adequate hydration, can aid in recovery and muscle protein synthesis.

- **Personalized Guidance:** Working with a registered dietitian or nutritionist experienced in sports nutrition is highly recommended when following the carnivore diet with the goal to maximize athletic performance. These professionals can provide personalized guidance based on individual needs, goals, and training demands. They can help assess nutrient requirements, design meal plans, and address any potential nutrient deficiencies or performance-related concerns.

• **Individuality Factor:** It's important to note that the carnivore diet may not be suitable for all athletes or individuals with high energy demands. Some individuals may find it extremely challenging to meet their energy needs without an adequate intake of carbohydrates, which are the primary fuel source for intense physical activities.

In all cases, it is important to prioritize overall health, performance, and long-term sustainability when considering any dietary approach, including the carnivore diet. Regular monitoring of performance, energy levels, and overall well-being is essential to assess the effectiveness and suitability of a specific dietary approach in supporting an individual's athletic goals. By closely monitoring these factors, individuals can gain insights into how their body is responding to the chosen diet and make any necessary adjustments to optimize their performance and well-being.

8. How Does the Carnivore Diet Impact Blood Sugar Control?

The effects of the carnivore diet on blood sugar control can vary among individuals, but typically the carnivore diet has a positive impact on blood sugar management, particularly for those with insulin resistance or diabetes.

Here are some key factors to consider regarding the carnivore diet's influence on blood sugar control:

- **Carbohydrate Elimination:** The carnivore diet eliminates most, if not all, sources of carbohydrates, including grains, fruits, vegetables, nuts, seeds, and legumes. By minimizing carbohydrate intake, the body enters a state of ketosis, where it relies on fat as its primary fuel source instead of glucose derived from carbohydrates. This shift in fuel metabolism can lead to improved blood sugar control in individuals who are insulin resistant or have difficulty regulating their blood sugar levels.

- **Stable Blood Sugar Levels:** With reduced carbohydrate intake, the carnivore diet may result in fewer fluctuations in blood sugar levels throughout the day. By avoiding high-glycemic carbohydrates that can cause rapid spikes in blood sugar, individuals may experience more stable and controlled blood sugar levels, potentially reducing the need for insulin or other blood sugar-lowering medications, such as Metformin (Glucophage®).

- **Individual Responses:** It's important to note that individual responses to the carnivore diet's impact on blood sugar control can vary. Factors such as metabolic health, insulin sensitivity, activity levels, and overall health status play an important role in determining how blood sugar levels will be influenced. Some individuals may experience significant improvements in blood sugar control, while others may not see substantial changes. Regular monitoring of blood sugar levels and consultation with healthcare professionals are crucial to assess individual responses and make necessary adjustments to medication dosages, if needed.

• **Medication Adjustments:** Individuals with diabetes or those using blood sugar-lowering medications (i.e. sulfonylureas) should work closely with healthcare professionals, such as endocrinologists or registered dietitians, when implementing the carnivore diet. As carbohydrate intake is significantly reduced, medication dosages may need to be adjusted to avoid hypoglycemia (low blood sugar). Regular blood sugar monitoring and close communication with healthcare providers are essential to ensure safe and effective blood sugar management while following the carnivore diet.

It's important to note that using the carnivore diet for therapeutic purposes may not be necessary for all individuals, especially those without insulin resistance, diabetes, or other metabolic problems. Carbohydrates are a crucial energy source for the body, and individuals engaging in intense physical activities or those with specific health conditions may require a more balanced dietary approach that includes healthy, whole-food sources of carbohydrates.

9. Are There Any Potential Psychological or Social Implications of Following the Carnivore Diet?

The psychological and social implications of following the carnivore diet can vary among individuals and may have an impact on mental well-being and social interactions. It is important to consider these aspects when evaluating the suitability of the carnivore diet for your lifestyle and overall health:

• **Feelings of Isolation:** The carnivore diet, with its restriction of plant-based foods, can lead to feelings of isolation or exclusion in social situations where food choices are limited. Sharing meals and participating in social gatherings may become challenging, as the diet does not align with typical social norms and eating patterns. This can result in individuals feeling disconnected from their social circles or experiencing a sense of being different.

• **Limited Food Choices:** The restrictive nature of the carnivore diet, which eliminates entire food groups (99.99% of plants), may contribute to a sense of deprivation or monotony in food choices. Restrictive diets can increase the focus on food, leading to heightened cravings and potential obsessions with food or eating behaviors. This can impact the psychological well-being of individuals and potentially contribute to disordered eating patterns.

- **Unhealthy Relationship with Food**: Strict dietary rules and the emphasis on eliminating entire food groups may contribute to an unhealthy relationship with food. Some individuals may develop a mindset of "good" and "bad" foods, leading to feelings of guilt or anxiety when deviating from the prescribed diet. This can create a rigid and unsustainable approach to eating, potentially impacting mental well-being and overall quality of life.

- **Nutritional Concerns:** The restrictive nature of the carnivore diet raises concerns about potential nutrient deficiencies, which can also impact mental health. Nutrients such as certain vitamins, minerals, trace elements, fiber, and beneficial phytochemicals found in plant-based foods have been associated with mental well-being and the prevention of mental health disorders. Excluding these nutrients from the diet may potentially increase the risk of nutrient imbalances that could affect mood, cognition, and overall mental well-being.

- **Support and Guidance:** Individuals following the carnivore diet should prioritize mental well-being and seek support from healthcare professionals, such as registered dietitians or therapists, who specialize in disordered eating or psychological aspects of nutrition. These professionals can provide guidance, support, and help individuals navigate the psychological challenges associated with dietary restrictions. Additionally, connecting with online communities or support groups of individuals following similar dietary patterns can provide a sense of belonging and shared experiences. It is crucial to strike a balance between dietary choices and overall well-being.

Prioritizing mental health, establishing a positive relationship with food, and seeking support when needed are essential factors for individuals following the carnivore diet or any restrictive eating pattern. Collaborating with healthcare professionals who can provide personalized guidance can help individuals navigate the psychological and social implications associated with restrictive dietary approaches, including the carnivore diet.

10. Is the Carnivore Diet Suitable for Everyone?

The carnivore diet, like any dietary approach, is not suitable for everyone. There are several factors to consider when determining the appropriateness of the carnivore diet for an individual, including:

• **Medical Conditions:** Individuals with certain medical conditions should exercise caution or even avoid the carnivore diet altogether. For example, individuals with kidney disease may need to limit their protein intake, as excessive protein can put additional strain on the kidneys. People with certain metabolic disorders, such as porphyria, may also need to avoid high-protein diets. Individuals with such medical conditions must consult with healthcare professionals or registered dietitians who can provide personalized guidance and recommendations tailored to their specific health needs. Taking into account individual health concerns and seeking professional advice can help ensure the safety and appropriateness of a particular diet.

- **Pregnancy and Breastfeeding:** The carnivore diet may not provide sufficient nutrients for the needs of both the mother and the developing baby during pregnancy and breastfeeding. It is essential to ensure an adequate intake of key nutrients, including folate, iron, zinc, calcium, potassium, magnesium, vitamin C, and omega-3 fatty acids, many of which are found in plant-based foods. Pregnant or breastfeeding women should consult with healthcare professionals to develop a well-rounded and balanced eating plan that supports their increased nutritional requirements.

- **Individual Nutrient Requirements:** Each person has unique nutrient requirements based on factors such as age, sex, activity level, and overall health status. While the carnivore diet can provide a wide range of essential nutrients, careful consideration should be given to ensure an adequate intake of specific nutrients that may be lacking, such as fiber, vitamin C, certain minerals (i.e. potassium, magnesium, etc), and phytonutrients found in plant-based foods. Regular monitoring of nutrient status through blood tests and consultations with healthcare professionals or registered dietitians is advisable to address any potential nutrient deficiencies.

- **Personalization and Variations:** The carnivore diet can be personalized and adapted to suit individual needs and goals. Some individuals may find that a modified version of the carnivore diet, which includes limited amounts of plant-based foods, such as certain fruits and vegetables, better meets their nutritional requirements and supports overall health. Generally, it is important to be flexible and listen to your own body's cues, making adjustments if necessary.

11. Can the Carnivore Diet Be Sustainable for the Environment?

The environmental sustainability of the carnivore diet is a complex issue that requires consideration of various factors. While the diet itself emphasizes animal-based foods, it is important to recognize the potential environmental impact associated with the production and consumption of animal foods in very large quantities. Here are some important key points about this topic to consider:

- **Greenhouse Gas Emissions:** Animal agriculture, particularly the production of ruminant animals like cattle, is a significant contributor to greenhouse gas emissions, primarily in the form of methane. Methane is a potent greenhouse gas that contributes to climate change. Reducing the overall consumption of animal products, including meat, can help mitigate these emissions.

- **Land Use and Deforestation:** Livestock farming requires significant land resources for grazing and feed production. The expansion of agricultural land, often achieved through deforestation, can lead to habitat destruction and loss of biodiversity. Choosing meats from sustainable farming practices that prioritize regenerative agriculture and minimize land use impacts can help reduce the environmental footprint.

- **Water Consumption and Pollution:** Animal agriculture requires substantial water resources, both for livestock hydration and crop irrigation. Additionally, intensive farming practices can lead to water pollution through the release of animal waste and the use of chemical fertilizers and pesticides, which can contaminate nearby water sources. Supporting farming systems that implement responsible water management practices can help mitigate these impacts.

- **Alternative Protein Sources:** Exploring alternative protein sources, such as sustainably-sourced seafood, can help diversify the diet and reduce the environmental burden associated with animal agriculture.

- **Sustainable Sourcing:** When choosing animal-based foods, individuals can prioritize sourcing from local, organic, and regenerative farms that follow sustainable practices. These farms often focus on animal welfare, environmental stewardship, and ecosystem restoration, contributing to a more sustainable food system.

It is worth noting that the environmental impact of any diet extends beyond the food choices themselves. Factors such as food waste, packaging, transportation, and food system inefficiencies also play a significant role. Adopting sustainable practices beyond dietary choices, such as reducing food waste, supporting local and seasonal produce, and minimizing packaging, can further contribute to environmental sustainability.

In conclusion, while the carnivore diet's heavy reliance on animal-based foods can raise some concerns about its environmental sustainability, individuals following the diet can take steps to minimize their impact. This includes selecting meats from sustainable farming practices, diversifying protein sources, and considering the broader environmental implications of their dietary choices.

12. Can Children Follow the Carnivore Diet?

Childhood is a crucial phase characterized by rapid growth, development, and the establishment of lifelong habits. During this period, providing children with a nutritionally balanced diet is essential to support their overall health, immune function, and cognitive development. While the carnivore diet emphasizes nutrient-dense, bioavailable, animal-based foods, completely excluding fruits, vegetables, nuts, seeds, and other plant-based foods may have negative implications for children's nutrient intake and long-term health. Here are some important key points to consider:

- **Micronutrient Deficiencies:** Fruits and vegetables are rich sources of essential vitamins, minerals, trace elements, and beneficial phytonutrients (i.e. carotenoids, ellagic acid, flavonoids, resveratrol, etc), which are very important for children's growth and development. For example, fruits are excellent sources of vitamin C, folate, and potassium, while vegetables provide essential vitamins A, K, and various minerals and trace elements. Excluding these food groups may increase the risk of nutrient deficiencies in children, potentially compromising their immune system function, bone health, development, and overall well-being.

- **Fiber Intake:** Plant-based foods are significant sources of dietary fiber. Fiber plays a vital role in maintaining digestive health, preventing constipation, and regulating blood sugar levels. Without sufficient fiber, children may experience digestive issues and an increased risk of chronic diseases later in life, such as obesity, cardiovascular disease, and certain types of cancer.

- **Phytochemicals and Antioxidants:** Fruits, vegetables, nuts, seeds, whole grains, and legumes contain various phytochemicals and antioxidants, which have been associated with numerous health benefits. Examples include carotenoids, flavonoids, phenolic acids, glucosinolates, phytosterols, terpenes, polyphenols, etc. These compounds possess potent antioxidant, anti-inflammatory, and immune-boosting properties, providing protection against chronic diseases and promoting overall health. Excluding these foods from the diet may deprive children of the potential health benefits associated with these plant-derived bioactive compounds.

- **Carbohydrate and Fat Balance:** Children require a balanced intake of carbohydrates and fats for energy and growth. While animal-based foods in the carnivore diet can provide ample protein and fats, they may not offer the same variety and balance of nutrients found in plant-based foods. Complex carbohydrates from whole grains, fruits, and vegetables serve as a vital energy source for children's active lifestyles and support brain function.

- **Psychological and Social Considerations:** In addition to the nutritional aspects, it is crucial to consider the psychological and social implications of restricting a child's diet to only animal-based foods. Excluding entire food groups may lead to feelings of restriction, social isolation, and potentially unhealthy relationships with food. Encouraging a positive and balanced approach to eating, including a wide variety of nutrient-dense foods (both plant-based and animal-based), can support children's overall well-being and foster a healthier relationship with food.

Given all these factors, it is advisable to consult with pediatric healthcare professionals and registered dietitians who specialize in pediatric nutrition to ensure that children receive a balanced and age-appropriate diet. These experts can assess individual nutritional needs, provide guidance on food selection, portion sizes, and meal planning, and monitor children's growth and development to ensure optimal nutrition and overall health.

Overall, the carnivore diet is generally not recommended for children due to the potential risk of nutrient deficiencies and the importance of providing a well-rounded, balanced diet to support their growth and development. Collaborating with healthcare professionals and registered dietitians who specialize in pediatric nutrition is crucial for ensuring children's nutritional needs are being met for their optimal health and well-being.

13. How to Manage Social Situations and Eating Out While on the Carnivore Diet?

Managing social situations and eating out while following the carnivore diet may present some challenges. However, with careful planning and communication, it is possible to navigate these situations successfully. Here are some strategies to consider:

• **Research and Plan Ahead:** Before dining out, take the time to research restaurants or menu options that align with the carnivore diet. Many establishments now provide their menus online, which allows you to identify meat-centric dishes or customizable options. Look for restaurants that offer a variety of animal-based proteins, such as steakhouses, seafood restaurants, or barbecue joints.

- **Contact Restaurants in Advance:** If you are unsure about the availability of carnivore-friendly options at a specific restaurant, consider calling ahead or sending an email to inquire about their ability to accommodate your dietary preferences. Communicate your needs clearly and politely, and ask if they can modify dishes or provide alternative options to suit your requirements.

- **Focus on Simple Meat-Based Dishes:** When dining out, prioritize meat-based dishes as the foundation of your meal. Opt for cuts of meat like steak, chicken, pork, or fish, prepared with minimal seasoning or sauces. Requesting modifications, such as omitting sauces, dressings, or side dishes that are not carnivore-friendly, can help you tailor your meal to fit your dietary needs.

- **Bring Portable Carnivore-Friendly Snacks:** To ensure you have something to eat in social situations where carnivore-friendly options may be limited, consider bringing your own portable snacks. This could include jerky, liver chips, hard-boiled eggs, canned fish, or cheese. Having these snacks on hand can help you stay satiated and on track.

- **Host Gatherings or Potlucks:** If you find it challenging to follow the carnivore diet when attending social events, consider hosting gatherings or potlucks where you have control over the menu. This allows you to prepare carnivore-friendly dishes that you and your guests can enjoy. You can focus on meat-based main courses and encourage others to bring side dishes or salads that can accommodate both carnivore and non-carnivore preferences.

Apart from these tips, open communication and a flexible mindset are key when managing social situations and eating out on the carnivore diet. Inform your friends and family about your dietary choices in a respectful manner, and be willing to answer questions and provide explanations, if necessary. By planning ahead and being prepared, you can navigate social settings while staying true to the carnivore diet much easier.

14. Can the Carnivore Diet Cause Constipation?

The carnivore diet is inherently low in dietary fiber as it eliminates all plant-based foods, which are typically rich sources of fiber. Fiber is a type of non-nutritive carbohydrate that passes through the digestive system relatively intact and provides bulk to the stool, promoting regular bowel movements. Insufficient fiber intake can contribute to constipation or difficulty in passing stool.

Fiber plays several key important roles in maintaining optimal digestive health. It adds bulk to the stool, which helps stimulate the muscles in the digestive tract, facilitating the movement of waste through the intestines. Additionally, fiber can absorb water, softening the stool and easing its passage. Moreover, certain types of fiber act as prebiotics, serving as a food source for beneficial gut bacteria and supporting a healthier gut microbiome.

The low-fiber nature of the carnivore diet can potentially lead to constipation in some individuals. When dietary fiber is limited, the stool may become harder and drier, making it more difficult to pass. This can result in infrequent bowel movements and discomfort.

While the carnivore diet is low in fiber, there are strategies that individuals can employ to mitigate constipation:

- **Include Organ Meats:** Organ meats, such as liver and kidney, contain modest amounts of dietary fiber in addition to a wealth of essential micronutrients. Including these nutrient-dense foods in your diet may contribute to supporting digestive regularity and mitigating constipation symptoms.

- **Consume Bone Broth:** Bone broth, a nourishing and hydrating liquid derived from simmering animal bones and connective tissues, offers more than just flavor. It contains gelatin and collagen, which possess beneficial properties for gut health. These substances can help support the integrity of the gut lining and potentially improve bowel movements, aiding in the mitigation of constipation. Incorporating bone broth into the carnivore diet can provide an additional source of nutrients while potentially alleviating digestive discomfort.

- **Incorporate Low-Carb Vegetables:** Although the carnivore diet generally excludes vegetable consumption, individuals seeking to address constipation concerns may consider incorporating select low-carb options known for their gut-friendly properties. Leafy greens like spinach and kale, as well as cruciferous vegetables such as broccoli and cauliflower, can provide a modest amount of fiber while remaining consistent with a low-carbohydrate intake. These vegetables not only contribute to dietary variety but also offer potential relief from constipation by promoting regularity and supporting digestive health.

- **Stay Hydrated:** Drinking an adequate amount of water is essential for maintaining proper hydration and supporting regular bowel movements. Water helps soften the stool, making it easier to pass.

- **Consider Individual Variations:** It is important to note that individuals may vary in their sensitivity to low-fiber diets, and some people may experience minimal issues with constipation while following the carnivore diet. However, it is still advisable to monitor bowel movements and make necessary adjustments if needed.

- **Consult with Healthcare Professionals:** If constipation persists or becomes a significant concern while following the carnivore diet, it is recommended to consult with healthcare professionals, such as registered dietitians or gastroenterologists. These people can provide personalized recommendations, assess overall gut health, and suggest additional strategies or interventions to effectively alleviate constipation.

15. Is the Carnivore Diet Suitable for Individuals With Certain Medical Conditions?

Individuals with the following medical conditions should be careful about following the carnivore diet:

• **Kidney Disease:** The carnivore diet, which is naturally high in protein, may not be suitable for individuals with kidney disease. A high protein intake can put additional strain on the kidneys, potentially worsening kidney function. Moreover, the diet's low-fiber nature can further compromise kidney health, as fiber plays a role in reducing the risk of certain kidney complications. Individuals with kidney disease should work closely with healthcare professionals, such as nephrologists or registered dietitians, to develop a personalized dietary plan that considers their specific kidney function and nutritional needs. This ensures that their dietary choices are appropriate and supportive of their overall health condition.

• **Liver Disease:** Liver disease encompasses various conditions that affect the liver's structure or function. The carnivore diet's high intake of saturated fats and cholesterol, primarily derived from animal-based sources, may not be advisable for individuals with liver disease, especially those with conditions such as non-alcoholic fatty liver disease (NAFLD) or cirrhosis. These individuals often require dietary modifications that focus on reducing fat intake, promoting liver health, and managing associated conditions, such as insulin resistance or metabolic syndrome. Working with healthcare professionals or registered dietitians experienced in liver disease management is crucial for developing an appropriate dietary approach in such cases.

• **Metabolic Disorders:** Certain metabolic disorders, such as phenylketonuria (PKU) or maple syrup urine disease (MSUD), require strict dietary management to prevent the accumulation of specific amino acids or organic acids in the body. These disorders are known as inborn errors of metabolism and require specialized dietary approaches to ensure the proper management of the condition. The carnivore diet, with its emphasis on high protein intake, may not align with the dietary requirements of individuals with these conditions. Following a specialized medical diet, tailored to the individual's specific metabolic disorder, is essential for positive health outcomes. Healthcare professionals, including metabolic dietitians or metabolic specialists, should be consulted to design an appropriate dietary plan in such cases.

Overall, it is important to recognize that each medical condition is unique, and dietary recommendations should be tailored to the individual's specific needs. While the carnivore diet may not be suitable for individuals with certain medical conditions, other dietary approaches, such as modified versions of the ketogenic diet or therapeutic diets specific to the condition, may be more appropriate. Consulting with healthcare professionals or registered dietitians who specialize in a particular medical condition is crucial for developing a safe and effective therapeutic dietary plan.

Additionally, considerations for nutrient balance should also be taken into account. Individuals with certain medical conditions may have increased nutrient requirements or specific nutrient restrictions. The rigid nutritional composition of the carnivore diet may pose challenges in meeting these requirements. In such cases, personalized supplementation or targeted nutrient modifications may be necessary to ensure optimal nutritional status while adhering to the diet.

16. Is the Carnivore Diet Beneficial for Weight Loss?

Yes. The carnivore diet has shown great potential for weight loss, which is something that can be attributed to several factors. Firstly, the high-protein content of the diet promotes satiety and reduces appetite, leading to decreased calorie intake. Protein, as a macronutrient, has a higher thermic effect compared to carbohydrates and fats, which means that the body expends more energy to digest and process it compared to other macronutrients, resulting in a higher metabolic rate.

Secondly, by eliminating processed foods, added sugars, and refined carbohydrates, the carnivore diet naturally reduces calorie-dense, inflammatory, and nutritionally-poor foods, which contribute to weight gain, inflammation, and fluid retention. Lastly, the low-carbohydrate nature of the carnivore diet leads to a decrease in insulin levels, facilitating the breakdown of stored body fat for energy. Low insulin levels create a favorable environment for weight loss.

However, it is always important to consider overall caloric intake and energy balance when using the carnivore diet for weight loss. Weight loss occurs when there is a sustained energy deficit, with calorie expenditure exceeding calorie intake. Despite the satiating effect of protein, overeating on the carnivore diet can still lead to weight gain. Thus, mindful portion control and monitoring overall energy intake are crucial to ensure a calorie deficit for successful weight loss.

When considering the carnivore diet for weight loss, long-term sustainability and adherence must always be taken into account. The diet's restrictive nature, with the elimination of all plant-based foods, may pose challenges for some individuals to maintain over an extended period. For that reason, it is important to evaluate the practicality and personal preferences regarding food choices to ensure long-term adherence.

17. Does the Carnivore Diet Have Side Effects?

While many individuals report positive outcomes on the carnivore diet, it is important to also be aware of its potential side effects. These may include:

• **Digestive Changes:** Some individuals may experience digestive changes when transitioning to the carnivore diet. This may include temporary symptoms, such as bloating, gas, or changes in bowel movements. These changes are often attributed to the elimination of fiber-rich plant foods, which play a role in promoting regular bowel movements and maintaining gut health. Gradually adapting to the diet and including easily-digestible animal-based foods, like bone broth or organ meats can help alleviate these symptoms. Bone broth is an easily-digestible animal-based beverage rich in amino acids, fatty acids, electrolytes, vitamins, minerals, trace elements, collagen, and gelatin. Organ meats tend to have a softer texture and are more tender compared to other cuts of meat.

• **Altered Bowel Movements:** Due to the low-fiber nature of the carnivore diet, individuals may experience changes in bowel movements, including a decrease in stool frequency or firmer stools. However, it is important to note that individual responses may vary, and some individuals may not experience any changes in bowel movements at all. Ensuring adequate hydration and incorporating foods like bone broth can help alleviate constipation and support digestive regularity.

- **Changes in Cholesterol Levels:** The carnivore diet's high intake of animal-based fats and proteins, including saturated fats, may lead to changes in cholesterol levels. Some individuals may experience an increase in total cholesterol, LDL cholesterol ("bad" cholesterol), and HDL cholesterol ("good" cholesterol). However, it is important to interpret these changes in the context of overall cardiovascular health. For some individuals, the carnivore diet may lead to favorable changes in cholesterol particle size and distribution, which may be associated with a lower risk of heart disease. Regular monitoring of cholesterol levels and working with healthcare professionals can help assess individual risk factors and make informed decisions.

- **Micronutrient Deficiencies:** The elimination of plant-based foods in the carnivore diet can increase the risk of certain micronutrient deficiencies, such as vitamins C and E, potassium, magnesium, and antioxidants. These nutrients are predominantly found in fruits, vegetables, nuts, seeds, legumes, and whole grains. To mitigate potential deficiencies, individuals on the carnivore diet should consider incorporating nutrient-dense organ meats, seafood, eggs, full-fat dairy, and other animal-based products that provide a wide array of essential micronutrients. Additionally, targeted supplementation or periodic monitoring of nutritional status may be necessary to ensure adequate nutrient intake.

- **Long-Term Health Risks:** The long-term health risks associated with the carnivore diet are still not well understood. The high intake of saturated fats and cholesterol, if not balanced with other health-promoting factors, such as an active lifestyle, proper hydration, adequate sleep, and stress management, may increase the risk of certain health conditions, such as cardiovascular disease and certain types of cancer. For that reason, it is important to approach the carnivore diet with awareness and consider individual health factors, such as pre-existing health conditions, family history, and metabolic health. Regular monitoring of biomarkers, consultations with healthcare professionals, and personalized modifications to the diet can help mitigate potential long-term risks.

It is worth noting that individual responses to the carnivore diet can vary significantly. While some individuals may thrive on the diet, others may experience adverse effects. Thus, it is crucial to listen to your body, monitor health biomarkers, and seek guidance from healthcare professionals or registered dietitians to ensure that the carnivore diet is suitable for your individual circumstances.

Overall, understanding and addressing potential side effects, regular monitoring of health markers, and personalized adjustments to the diet are essential actions for optimizing the safety, effectiveness, and sustainability of the carnivore diet.

18. Can the Carnivore Diet Cause Nutrient Excesses?

While the carnivore diet can provide several important key nutrients, excessive intake of certain nutrients, such as vitamin A, iron, saturated fats, cholesterol, sodium, and omega-6 fatty acids, can be a concern in some cases and for some individuals. It is important to prioritize quality sources of animal-based foods, opt for the right cuts of meat, incorporate a variety of animal proteins, and consider periodic blood tests to monitor lipid profiles and ensure a balanced nutrient intake. Here is a list of potential nutrient excesses when following the carnivore diet:

• **Saturated Fats and Cholesterol:** The carnivore diet, which emphasizes animal-based foods, can lead to a higher than normal intake of saturated fats and dietary cholesterol. Excessive consumption of saturated fats has been associated with an increased risk of cardiovascular disease, while high cholesterol levels in the blood can contribute to plaque formation in the arteries. It is important to prioritize quality sources of animal-based foods, such as grass-fed or pasture-raised meats, which tend to have a more favorable fatty acid profile (omega-3s > omega-6s). Opting for leaner cuts of meat and incorporating a variety of animal proteins, including eggs, poultry, fish, and seafood, can help moderate the intake of saturated fats and cholesterol.

- **Iron:** Animal-based foods, especially red meats and organ meats, are rich sources of heme iron. While iron is an essential nutrient, excessive iron intake can be harmful, particularly for individuals with conditions like hereditary hemochromatosis or other iron-overload disorders. Regular monitoring of iron levels through blood tests is advisable for individuals on the carnivore diet, especially those consuming high amounts of iron-rich foods.

- **Vitamin A:** Organ meats, such as liver, are potent sources of vitamin A. While vitamin A is essential for various biological functions in the body, excessive intake of preformed vitamin A (retinol) from animal sources can lead to toxicity, known as hypervitaminosis A. Symptoms of hypervitaminosis A can include nausea, dizziness, hair loss, and bone abnormalities. Moderation and variety in animal protein sources can help avoid excessive vitamin A intake.

- **Sodium:** The carnivore diet, particularly when relying on processed or cured meats, may contribute to a higher sodium intake. Excessive sodium intake can increase the risk of high blood pressure and cardiovascular disease. It is important to be mindful of the sodium content of foods and prioritize fresh, unprocessed meats whenever possible. Balancing sodium with enough water, potassium intake, appropriate seasoning, and avoiding excessive or any salt in cooking may also help manage sodium levels.

- **Omega-6 Fatty Acids:** While animal-based foods can provide essential omega-3 fatty acids, such as EPA and DHA, the carnivore diet may lead to an imbalance in the ratio of omega-3s to omega-6s in the body. Excessive consumption of omega-6 fatty acids, mainly derived from grain-fed and processed meats, can promote inflammation. Incorporating omega-3-rich sources, such as fatty fish (i.e. salmon, mackerel, sardines, etc) or supplementation with high-quality fish oil, can help restore a healthier balance between these essential fatty acids.

It is important to note that individual nutrient needs and tolerances can vary. Regular monitoring of blood lipid profiles, iron levels, and other relevant biomarkers is recommended to assess individual nutrient status and prevent potential nutrient excesses. Consulting with healthcare professionals or registered dietitians who specialize in low-carb diets can provide personalized guidance on nutrient intake, supplementation, and ensuring a balanced approach to nutrition.

19. Can the Carnivore Diet Cause Digestive Issues?

Some individuals may experience digestive issues when transitioning to the carnivore diet, such as constipation or changes in bowel movements. This can be attributed to the sudden elimination of fiber-rich foods commonly found in plant-based sources. Adequate hydration, consumption of fatty cuts of meat, and gradually adjusting the diet may help alleviate these issues.

However, if digestive problems persist or worsen, it is recommended to seek medical advice. Here are some important key points to consider about the emergence of digestive issues on the carnivore diet:

- **Constipation:** The low-fiber nature of the carnivore diet can contribute to constipation for some individuals. Fiber plays a crucial role in promoting regular bowel movements by adding bulk to the stool and aiding in its passage through the digestive tract. The absence of fiber from plant-based sources in the carnivore diet may result in reduced stool volume and slower bowel transit time. To alleviate constipation, it is important to focus on alternative sources of dietary fiber, such as organ meats (small amounts of animal-based fiber), bone broth, or even low-carb vegetables (i.e. leafy greens, cruciferous vegetables, zucchini, etc) that can be utilized within the context of a low-carb, meat-based diet. These foods can provide some fiber and promote better bowel movements. Additionally, adequate hydration is also essential to support regularity and soften the stool.

- **Changes in Bowel Movements:** Transitioning to the carnivore diet can lead to changes in bowel movements, such as a decrease in frequency or alterations in stool consistency. These changes may be attributed to the altered composition of the diet, reduced fiber intake, and changes in gut microbiota. It is important to allow time for the body to adapt to the new dietary pattern. Gradually transitioning to the carnivore diet and ensuring sufficient hydration through filtered water and electrolyte-rich beverages (i.e. bone broth, raw milk, electrolyte-infused water), can help mitigate these changes. Additionally, monitoring bowel movements and seeking medical advice if issues persist or worsen is advisable.

- **Gut Microbiota:** The carnivore diet's impact on the gut microbiota, which plays a crucial role in digestive health, is an area of ongoing research. The reduction or elimination of plant-based foods can affect the diversity and composition of gut bacteria. While some individuals report improvements in digestive symptoms due to the elimination of potentially irritating plant foods, the long-term effects of the carnivore diet on overall gut health are not well-understood. To support a healthier gut microbiome while following the carnivore diet, it is important to prioritize gut health by incorporating well-sourced fermented foods, such as organic goat's milk yogurt or kefir, which provide beneficial bacteria (probiotics). Probiotic supplementation from reputable brands may also be considered to promote a more favorable gut microbiota environment.

- **Individual Variability:** It is essential to recognize that individual responses to the carnivore diet can vary. Some individuals may experience improved digestive function, while others may encounter challenges. Factors such as pre-existing digestive conditions, genetic predispositions, and overall dietary history can influence individual responses. It is recommended to monitor digestive symptoms and seek medical advice if issues persist or if there are specific concerns about digestive health.

- **Medical Advice:** If you experience persistent or severe digestive issues while following the carnivore diet, it may be necessary to seek medical advice. Consulting with healthcare professionals or registered dietitians who specialize in digestive health can provide personalized guidance, assess potential underlying causes, and recommend appropriate interventions to address any existing digestive issues.

20. Does the Carnivore Diet Increase the Risk of Cardiovascular Disease?

The carnivore diet's influence on cardiovascular health is a topic of ongoing research and discussion. While the diet eliminates processed foods and refined carbohydrates, which are commonly associated with an increased risk of cardiovascular disease (CVD), it is important to consider other factors that may affect cardiovascular health, such as saturated fat and cholesterol intake. Here are some important key points to consider about the carnivore diet's impact on cardiovascular health:

- **Saturated Fat:** The carnivore diet typically includes a high intake of saturated fats from animal sources, including fatty cuts of meat, butter, and other animal fats. High saturated fat intake has traditionally been linked to an increased risk of CVD. Saturated fats can raise low-density lipoprotein (LDL) cholesterol levels, commonly referred to as "bad" cholesterol, which is associated with an increased risk of cardiovascular disease. However, recent research has questioned the direct link between saturated fat intake and cardiovascular disease, suggesting that other factors, such as overall diet quality and individual metabolic responses, also play a significant role.

- **Cholesterol:** Animal-based foods are a significant source of dietary cholesterol. While dietary cholesterol has less of an impact on blood cholesterol levels compared to saturated fat, it is still a consideration for cardiovascular health. The relationship between dietary cholesterol and blood cholesterol is a complex topic and can vary between individuals. Some people are more sensitive to dietary cholesterol (also known as "hyper-responders"), while others show minimal changes. Typically, the body tightly regulates cholesterol levels, and endogenous liver production can compensate for dietary intake or absence to some extent.

- **Individual Factors:** It is important to consider individual factors when assessing the impact of the carnivore diet on cardiovascular health. Each person may have a unique metabolic response to dietary fat and cholesterol, influenced by genetics, overall diet quality, physical activity levels, and other lifestyle factors. Some individuals may experience an increase in LDL cholesterol levels when following the carnivore diet, while others may not.

- **Other Health Markers:** When evaluating cardiovascular health, it is important to consider other markers beyond cholesterol levels. Factors such as blood pressure, inflammation, insulin sensitivity, and oxidative stress play crucial roles in CVD development. While limited research is available, some studies have suggested potential benefits of the carnivore diet on these markers, such as improved insulin sensitivity and reduced inflammation, which can be beneficial for cardiovascular health.

- **Long-Term Effects:** Long-term studies assessing the effects of the carnivore diet on cardiovascular health are currently lacking. Most existing research is based on short-term studies or anecdotal evidence. Long-term sustainability and adherence to the carnivore diet, as well as the potential impact on overall dietary quality and nutrient intake, should be considered when evaluating its effects on cardiovascular health.

In summary, the carnivore diet's impact on cardiovascular disease risk is still being explored, and further research is needed to fully understand its long-term effects. While the diet eliminates processed foods and refined carbohydrates (which are inflammatory and impair metabolic health), it is very high in saturated fats and cholesterol.

Individual responses to saturated fats and cholesterol intake can vary, and other factors, such as overall diet quality and individual metabolic responses, may also play a role in determining cardiovascular risk. Thus, it is important to monitor cardiovascular health markers, such as blood lipid profiles and blood pressure, and to consult with healthcare professionals for personalized guidance on diet and cardiovascular risk management.

21. Does the Carnivore Diet Increase Testosterone?

Testosterone is a steroid hormone primarily associated with male sexual development and reproductive function. It also plays a crucial role in various physiological processes in the body, including muscle growth, bone density, and mood regulation. While the carnivore diet is often touted as a means to optimize testosterone levels, it is important to approach such claims with some consideration.

The carnivore diet, which emphasizes animal-based foods, provides a rich source of protein, healthy fats, and various essential micronutrients that are crucial for hormone production, including testosterone. Protein is particularly important as it provides the necessary amino acids for testosterone synthesis. However, it is worth noting that excessive protein intake does not necessarily equate to higher testosterone levels, as other factors also influence hormone production.

Maintaining an appropriate energy balance is particularly important for optimal testosterone levels. Severe calorie restriction or excessive energy deficits, which may occur on certain versions of the carnivore diet, can lead to decreased testosterone production. For that reason, it is crucial to ensure sufficient calorie intake to support hormone production and overall health.

Similarly to low-carbohydrate diets, the carnivore diet may lead to weight loss due to reduced calorie intake and the positive metabolic effects of carbohydrate restriction. Weight loss itself can have a positive impact on testosterone levels, as excess body fat is associated with lower testosterone production. Excessive adipose tissue (body fat) can contribute to increased production of the enzyme aromatase. Aromatase converts testosterone (a predominantly male hormone) into estrogen (a predominantly female hormone). This may lead to hormone imbalances, with relatively higher estrogen and lower testosterone levels. Achieving and maintaining a leaner body composition can help improve testosterone levels because lower levels of body fat are associated with reduced aromatase activity.

It's worth noting here that weight loss and changes in body composition can be achieved through various dietary approaches, and the carnivore diet is just one of them.

Testosterone levels are influenced by a wide range of factors, including genetics, age, lifestyle, stress levels, sleep quality, and underlying health conditions. Each individual may respond differently to dietary interventions, and some may experience more significant changes in their testosterone levels compared to others.

Currently, there is limited scientific research specifically examining the impact of the carnivore diet on testosterone levels. Most studies investigating the effects of diet on testosterone focus on macronutrient composition, rather than specific dietary patterns, such as the carnivore diet. Therefore, it is challenging to draw definitive conclusions about the diet's direct influence on testosterone

22. Can You Build Muscle on the Carnivore Diet?

Building muscle on the carnivore diet is very achievable, given its emphasis on high-quality animal-based protein sources that provide the necessary amino acids for muscle protein synthesis. Adequate protein intake, combined with resistance training and appropriate calorie intake, are prerequisites for muscle growth. On top of that, individual factors such as training intensity, overall calorie balance, and genetics also play a significant role in muscle development. Here are some important key points to consider about the carnivore diet's impact on muscle growth:

• **Protein Intake:** The carnivore diet is rich in animal-based protein, such as meat, fish, poultry, eggs, and dairy. These foods provide complete protein containing all essential amino acids necessary for muscle protein synthesis. Adequate protein intake is crucial for muscle growth and repair. The recommended protein intake for individuals aiming to build muscle is generally around 1.6-2.2 grams of protein per kilogram (kg) of body weight per day.

• **Resistance Training:** To build muscle, it is essential to engage in regular resistance training exercises. Resistance exercises, such as weightlifting or bodyweight exercises, create a stimulus that triggers muscle adaptation and growth. By providing resistance to muscles, these exercises stimulate the breakdown and subsequent rebuilding of muscle tissue, leading to muscle hypertrophy.

• **Calorie Intake:** To support muscle growth, it is important to consume an appropriate amount of calories. The carnivore diet can provide sufficient calories, mainly through protein and fat sources. It is crucial to ensure that your calorie intake meets the energy demands of your training and supports muscle growth. Keep in mind that your individual calorie needs may vary based on factors such as age, sex, physical activity levels, health status, and overall metabolism.

• **Micronutrient Support:** While the carnivore diet can provide essential macronutrients, such as protein and fats, it is important to also ensure adequate intake of micronutrients for optimal muscle function, hormone balance, metabolism, and overall health. Nutrient-dense animal foods, such as red meat, organ meats, eggs, dairy, and seafood, can contribute to meeting your micronutrient needs very effectively. However, it may be necessary to consider targeted supplementation or consult with a healthcare professional or registered dietitian to address any potential nutrient gaps.

- **Individual Factors:** It is important to acknowledge that individual factors, such as genetics, training intensity, recovery, and overall lifestyle, also play a significant role in muscle development. Each person may respond differently to dietary and training interventions, thus finding the approach that works best for an individual's goals and needs is very important.

23. Does the Carnivore Diet Improve Sexual Performance?

The impact of the carnivore diet on sexual performance is not well studied, and individual experiences may vary. While a nutrient-dense diet that supports overall health can indirectly contribute to improved sexual function, it is important to note that sexual performance is influenced by many factors, including hormonal balance, electrolyte balance, psychological well-being, and cardiovascular health. Here are some important key points to consider about the carnivore diet's impact on sexual performance:

- **Nutrient Density and Overall Health:** The carnivore diet emphasizes nutrient-dense animal foods that provide essential nutrients for overall health. Adequate nutrient intake is important for maintaining optimal bodily functions, including sexual health. Nutrients like zinc, vitamin D, selenium, magnesium, and omega-3 fatty acids found in animal-based foods have been associated with aspects of sexual health. However, more research is needed to establish a direct link between the carnivore diet and sexual performance.

• **Hormonal Balance:** Hormonal balance, particularly testosterone levels, can influence sexual function in both men and women. While some studies suggest that sufficient protein intake and overall healthy nutrition can support testosterone production, the specific impact of the carnivore diet on hormonal balance and sexual performance is not well understood. Factors such as genetics, age, stress levels, physical activity, and lifestyle choices can also influence hormonal balance and sexual function.

• **Psychological Well-being:** Psychological factors, such as stress, anxiety, and self-confidence, can significantly affect sexual performance. While the carnivore diet may contribute to overall well-being and potentially alleviate certain health conditions that can impact sexual health, its direct influence on psychological factors related to sexual performance is unclear.

• **Cardiovascular Health:** Cardiovascular health plays a vital role in sexual function. The carnivore diet's potential impact on cardiovascular health is still a subject of debate, as animal-based diets are naturally high in saturated fats and cholesterol. While the elimination of processed foods and refined carbohydrates can have a positive effect on cardiovascular risk factors, the long-term implications of the carnivore diet on cardiovascular health and sexual performance require further investigation to make official statements.

- **Individual Factors:** It is important to recognize that sexual performance is influenced by numerous individual factors, including genetics, lifestyle, health status, relationship dynamics, and overall well-being. While dietary choices can contribute to overall health, they are just one aspect of the complex interplay of factors that affect sexual performance.

24. Does the Carnivore Diet Improve Body Composition?

The carnivore diet, combined with resistance training, can support improvements in body composition. By providing ample protein and essential micronutrients, it can help promote muscle growth and fat loss when combined with a calorie-appropriate approach. However, individual responses may vary, and it is important to monitor overall calorie intake and adjust the diet to meet specific fitness goals. Here are some important key points to consider about the carnivore diet's impact on body composition:

- **Adequate Protein Intake:** The carnivore diet emphasizes animal-based protein sources, which provide essential amino acids necessary for muscle protein synthesis. Adequate protein intake is crucial for building and maintaining lean muscle mass. Protein is also more satiating than carbohydrates or fats, which can help with appetite control and weight management.

- **Muscle Growth:** Resistance training is a key component in improving body composition. When combined with a diet that provides sufficient protein and overall energy balance, the carnivore diet can effectively promote muscle growth. Protein plays a vital role in repairing and building muscle tissue after exercise and serves as the building block for various hormones, including testosterone. Testosterone is an anabolic hormone that is important for muscle growth and development.

- **Fat Loss:** The carnivore diet, by eliminating processed foods, added sugars, and refined carbohydrates, can naturally reduce calorie intake and promote weight loss. Furthermore, a higher protein intake may increase satiety and help preserve muscle mass during calorie restriction, leading to a greater proportion of weight loss coming from fat rather than muscle tissue.

- **Caloric Balance:** While the carnivore diet can contribute to improvements in body composition, achieving the desired results also depends on caloric balance. Creating an appropriate calorie deficit or surplus based on individual goals is crucial. This involves monitoring overall energy intake and expenditure to support fat loss or muscle gain.

- **Individual Variability:** It is important to recognize that individual responses to the carnivore diet and its impact on body composition can vary. Factors such as genetics, age, sex, training status, and overall lifestyle play a significant role. Some individuals may respond well to the carnivore diet in terms of body composition, while others may require different dietary approaches for optimal results.

- **Sustainable Approach:** Long-term sustainability is essential for achieving and maintaining improvements in body composition, no matter what diet you follow. While the carnivore diet may provide short-term benefits, it is important to consider the long-term feasibility and potential nutrient deficiencies associated with the complete exclusion of plant-based foods. Adapting the carnivore diet to incorporate nutrient-dense organ meats, incorporating a variety of animal foods, and periodically reassessing nutrient status, are essential factors for long-term sustainability and results.

25. Does the Carnivore Diet Cause Kidney Problems?

The impact of the carnivore diet on kidney health is a hot topic of debate. While a high protein intake can increase the workload on the kidneys, there is limited scientific evidence linking the carnivore diet specifically to kidney problems in healthy individuals. However, those with pre-existing kidney conditions should exercise caution and consult with healthcare professionals before making significant dietary changes. Here are some important considerations about the carnivore diet's impact on kidney health:

• **Protein Intake:** The carnivore diet is naturally high in protein, as it emphasizes animal-based foods as its primary source of nutrition. High protein intake can increase the workload on the kidneys, as the kidneys are responsible for filtering out and excreting waste products generated from protein metabolism. The impact of protein on kidney function is influenced by various factors, including overall kidney health, hydration status, and individual tolerance.

• **Kidney Function:** In healthy individuals with normal kidney function, the kidneys are capable of adapting to a higher protein intake. They can adjust their filtration rate to accommodate the increased protein load. However, individuals with pre-existing kidney conditions, such as chronic kidney disease or kidney stones, may be more susceptible to potential adverse effects from a high-protein diet. These individuals should exercise caution and consult with healthcare professionals before making significant dietary changes, including adopting the carnivore diet.

• **Individual Variability:** It is important to recognize that individual responses to the carnivore diet and its impact on kidney health can vary. Factors such as age, sex, genetics, overall health status, and pre-existing kidney conditions play a significant role. Some individuals may tolerate a higher protein intake without experiencing any negative effects on kidney function, while others may be more susceptible to health complications.

- **Hydration and Electrolyte Balance:** Adequate hydration is crucial for maintaining kidney health, regardless of the diet followed. Consuming an adequate amount of fluids helps ensure optimal kidney function and the elimination of waste products. Additionally, electrolyte balance, particularly sodium and potassium, is important for maintaining proper physiological function. Sodium and potassium are two key electrolytes involved in various physiological processes within the body and play essential roles in maintaining cellular function, nerve transmission, and fluid balance.

- **Monitoring and Individualization:** Regular monitoring of kidney function, including blood tests to assess markers such as creatinine and urea nitrogen, can provide valuable information about kidney health. Consulting with healthcare professionals, such as nephrologists or registered dietitians, can help individuals with pre-existing kidney conditions navigate dietary choices and make appropriate modifications to ensure kidney health is prioritized.

26. How Long Does It Take to Adapt to the Carnivore Diet?

The length of adaptation to the carnivore diet can vary among individuals. Factors such as metabolic flexibility, previous dietary habits, overall health status, and individual physiology can influence the duration of the adaptation period. Some individuals may transition smoothly and adapt relatively quickly, while others may experience a longer adjustment phase.

During the adaptation period, it is common for individuals to experience digestive changes. This may include shifts in bowel movements, such as looser or firmer stools, as well as changes in gut microbiota composition. These changes occur as the digestive system adjusts to the different composition of the diet, which is devoid of fiber and contains a very high proportion of protein and animal-based foods.

It is not uncommon for individuals to also experience changes in energy levels during the adaptation phase. Some people report an initial decrease in energy, often referred to as the "low-carb flu" or "keto flu" as the body slowly adjusts to using fat as its primary fuel source. This can be attributed to the shift from relying on carbohydrates for energy to utilizing fat stores. However, energy levels usually stabilize as the body adapts to the new dietary pattern.

The adaptation period to the carnivore diet typically ranges from a few days to a few weeks. During this time, it is advisable to be patient and allow the body to adjust gradually. It is also important to listen to your body and make modifications if necessary. Gradually reintroducing certain foods or experimenting with different types of animal-based products can help identify individual tolerances and optimize the diet for long-term adherence.

27. What Supplements Should I Take While Following the Carnivore Diet?

While the carnivore diet can provide many essential nutrients, certain supplements can be beneficial to take. These may include omega-3 fatty acids (if not consuming adequate amounts of fatty fish), vitamin D (especially for individuals with limited sun exposure), and electrolytes (to support hydration, energy, and performance). Here are some important things to consider about supplementation while on the carnivore diet:

• **Omega-3 Fatty Acids:** The carnivore diet, if not properly designed, can lack beneficial omega-3 fatty acids, which are primarily found in fatty fish. Omega-3 fatty acids play important roles in cardiovascular health, brain function, joint health, and inflammation regulation. Individuals not consuming fatty fish regularly may consider supplementation with high-quality fish or krill oil, which provide high amounts of eicosapentaenoic acid (EPA) and docosahexaenoic acid (DHA), the bioavailable, active forms of omega-3s not found in the plant kingdom (i.e. chia seeds, flaxseeds, walnuts, hemp seeds, etc)

• **Vitamin D:** Vitamin D is synthesized in the skin upon exposure to sunlight. However, individuals with limited sun exposure, such as those living in northern latitudes or who have darker skin, may have insufficient levels of vitamin D. Since few food sources naturally contain vitamin D, supplementation may be necessary to maintain optimal levels. Consulting with a healthcare professional or registered dietician can help determine the appropriate dosage based on your individual needs and blood test results.

• **Electrolytes:** The carnivore diet, with its low carbohydrate intake, can cause increased water excretion and electrolyte loss. This may be particularly relevant during the adaptation phase or for individuals who partake in intense physical activity (i.e. HIIT, CrossFit, spinning/cycling, martial arts, etc). Supplementing with electrolytes, such as sodium, potassium, and magnesium, can help maintain proper electrolyte balance in the body and prevent dehydration.

• **Individualized Approach:** While these are some common supplements to consider on the carnivore diet, it is crucial to approach supplementation on an individual basis. Factors such as pre-existing health conditions, nutrient intake, gut health, and blood test results should also be taken into account. Consulting with a healthcare professional or registered dietitian who is knowledgeable about low-carb diets can help assess individual needs and provide personalized recommendations.

• **Monitoring and Adjustments:** It is important to periodically monitor nutrient status through blood tests to ensure that nutrient needs are being met and to guide supplementation decisions. Regular monitoring can help identify any potential deficiencies or imbalances that may require adjustments in the diet or supplementation routine.

28. Does the Carnivore Diet Affect Sleep Quality?

The specific impact of the carnivore diet on sleep is not extensively studied, and there is a lack of scientific evidence to support definitive conclusions. Overall, the relationship between the carnivore diet and sleep quality remains unclear.

Typically, a well-balanced diet that provides essential nutrients and supports overall health can indirectly contribute to better sleep. Nutrients like magnesium, zinc, and B vitamins found in animal-based foods are important for maintaining healthy sleep patterns. Additionally, a healthy body weight and reduced inflammation, which can be influenced by the carnivore diet, may positively impact sleep quality.

Sleep is a complex process influenced by various factors, including genetics, lifestyle, physical activity, stress levels, and sleep hygiene practices. Individual responses to dietary changes, including the carnivore diet, can vary significantly. Some individuals may experience improvements in sleep quality, while others may not notice any significant changes or even experience disruptions in sleep.

In addition to dietary factors, maintaining good sleep hygiene practices is particularly important for optimal sleep. This includes following a consistent sleep schedule, creating a conducive sleep environment, limiting exposure to electronic devices before bed, managing stress, and avoiding stimulants like caffeine or theobromine close to bedtime.

It is important to consider personal factors that may impact sleep quality. For example, some individuals may experience changes in energy levels or digestive patterns during the adaptation phase of the carnivore diet, which could potentially affect sleep. Monitoring these changes and making adjustments as needed can help optimize sleep quality.

Sleep is a multifaceted aspect of overall health, and addressing all aspects of well-being is essential for promoting healthy sleep. Alongside dietary choices, incorporating stress management techniques, regular physical activity, and addressing any underlying sleep disorders or medical conditions can all contribute to better sleep outcomes.

In summary, while the specific impact of the carnivore diet on sleep is not well-studied, maintaining a well-balanced diet that supports overall health and incorporating good sleep hygiene practices can positively influence sleep quality. Individual responses may vary, and it is essential to address personal factors that may affect sleep. Taking a holistic approach to health, including diet, lifestyle, and sleep habits, is very important for optimizing sleep quality.

29. Does the Carnivore Diet Make Your Body More Acidic?

The carnivore diet, characterized by a higher than normal consumption of animal-based foods, particularly high in protein, has the potential to increase acid production in the body. Protein metabolism results in the formation of sulfuric, phosphoric, and other organic acids, which can contribute to an acidic environment.

The body tightly regulates acid-base balance through various physiological mechanisms to maintain proper pH levels. These mechanisms include buffering systems, such as bicarbonate, and the elimination of excess acids through the kidneys and lungs. In healthy individuals, these processes generally maintain a relatively stable pH level, regardless of dietary choices.

Short-term consumption of animal protein, as is common in the carnivore diet, is unlikely to significantly alter overall pH levels or disrupt acid-base balance within the body. The body can effectively manage transient increases in acid production by activating buffering systems and excreting excess acids.

The impact of the carnivore diet on the body's acid-base balance may vary among individuals based on factors such as metabolic rate, kidney function, and overall health status. Some individuals may have a higher tolerance for increased acid load, while others may be more susceptible to disturbances in acid-base balance.

While the carnivore diet has the potential to temporarily increase acid production, it is important to emphasize that the body has mechanisms in place to regulate acid-base balance. Monitoring overall health, including kidney function and bone health, can provide valuable insights into the impact of diet on the body's acid-base balance. Consulting with healthcare professionals, such as registered dietitians or physicians, can help assess individual needs and address any concerns.

It is important to note that the overall dietary context, beyond just protein intake, can influence acid-base balance. For example, fruits and vegetables, which are excluded from the carnivore diet, are alkaline-forming foods that can help balance acidity in the body. However, it is possible to optimize acid-base balance within the confines of the carnivore diet by choosing high-quality animal-based foods and considering other potential alkalizing factors, such as mineral-rich bone broth or certain seasonings.

Overall, while the carnivore diet may lead to transient increases in acid production due to its high animal protein content, the body has natural mechanisms in place to maintain acid-base balance. Short-term consumption of animal protein doesn't significantly alter overall pH levels. Monitoring overall health and individual responses, as well as considering other dietary factors, can help ensure a balanced approach to acid-base homeostasis while following the carnivore diet.

30. Does the Carnivore Diet Impair Detoxification?

The carnivore diet, which emphasizes high-quality, bioavailable, animal-based foods, can provide essential nutrients that support various detoxification pathways in the body. These nutrients include B vitamins (e.g. vitamins B6, B12, and folate), zinc, selenium, and antioxidants (e.g. vitamins C and E). These substances are involved in enzymatic reactions necessary for the body's natural detoxification processes.

Detoxification in the body occurs through two main phases: Phase I and Phase II. Phase I involves the activation of enzymes that metabolize toxins, while Phase II involves conjugation reactions that facilitate the elimination of these metabolites. Nutrients found in animal-based foods, such as amino acids, vitamins, minerals, and trace elements, play vital roles in these processes.

The liver, a key organ involved in detoxification, relies on adequate nutrient intake to support its metabolic functions. The carnivore diet, when properly designed, can provide the necessary nutrients to support optimal liver function and detoxification. However, it is important to consider individual variations and potential nutrient deficiencies that may arise from excluding all plant-based foods completely.

Antioxidants found in animal-based foods, such as selenium, CoQ10, and vitamin E, can help protect against oxidative stress and support the body's detoxification pathways. These antioxidants neutralize free radicals generated during the detoxification process and reduce the risk of cellular damage.

The effectiveness of detoxification processes and nutrient utilization can vary among individuals due to factors such as genetics, overall health status, and exposure to toxins. Some individuals may have higher detoxification capacity, while others may be more susceptible to toxin accumulation. Consulting with healthcare professionals, such as registered dietitians or physicians, can help assess individual needs and provide personalized recommendations.

While meat can provide essential nutrients for detoxification, it is important to ensure a well-rounded nutrient intake. This may involve incorporating a wider range of nutrient-dense animal foods, such as organ meats, seafood, full-fat dairy, and eggs, while considering supplementation or periodic monitoring to address potential nutrient deficiencies. Additionally, individualized dietary and lifestyle factors should also be taken into account for optimal detoxification support.

31. Can the Carnivore Diet Cure Autoimmune Diseases?

Autoimmune diseases are characterized by an immune system that mistakenly attacks healthy cells and tissues in the body. These conditions are complex, chronic and multifactorial, involving genetic predisposition, environmental triggers, gut permeability, and dysregulation of the immune system.

While anecdotal reports suggest that some individuals may experience improvements in autoimmune symptoms when following the carnivore diet, official scientific evidence supporting its effectiveness in managing autoimmune diseases is currently limited. Research in this area is still in its early stages, and more rigorous studies are needed to evaluate the long-term effects and benefits.

Autoimmune diseases often require comprehensive treatment approaches that include medication, supplementation, lifestyle modifications, and dietary interventions. Nutritional factors play a significant role in managing autoimmune conditions, and a well-rounded diet that is anti-inflammatory and provides a wide range of nutrients is generally recommended.

Autoimmune diseases are highly individualized, and what works for one person may not work for another. The response to dietary interventions, including the carnivore diet, can vary greatly among individuals. Some individuals may experience improvements in symptoms, while others may not see any significant changes or even experience negative effects. It is crucial to consider individual health needs, medical history, and consult with healthcare professionals, such as immunologists, endocrinologists, rheumatologists, or registered dietitians, to develop a personalized treatment plan for managing autoimmunity.

The carnivore diet's exclusion of plant-based foods may limit the intake of certain compounds, such as antioxidants (i.e. vitamin C), phytochemicals (i.e. polyphenols, terpenoids, organosulfur compounds, etc), and fiber, which are important for immune health and overall well-being. Additionally, the high intake of animal-based foods, particularly processed meats, may have negative effects on inflammation and gut microbiota composition, which can influence autoimmune diseases. These factors should be carefully considered when evaluating the suitability of the carnivore diet for individuals with autoimmune conditions.

Managing autoimmune diseases requires a holistic and multifaceted approach that addresses multiple aspects of health, including nutrition, supplementation, stress management, sleep, physical activity, and medication. It is important to work with healthcare professionals who specialize in autoimmune diseases to develop an individualized treatment plan that considers all the unique needs and circumstances of each individual.

Overall, while some individuals report improvements in autoimmune symptoms when following the carnivore diet, the scientific evidence supporting its effectiveness in managing autoimmune diseases is currently limited. Autoimmune conditions are complex, and a comprehensive treatment approach that incorporates supplementation, medication, lifestyle modifications, and dietary interventions is typically recommended for successful health outcomes.

32. Is the Carnivore Diet Beneficial for Skin Health?

Skin health is influenced by a variety of factors, including genetics, lifestyle, environmental factors, and nutrition. A well-balanced diet that provides essential nutrients is crucial for maintaining healthy skin.

The specific impact of the carnivore diet on skin health is not extensively studied, and there is a lack of scientific evidence to support its effectiveness in improving or worsening skin conditions. Individual experiences may vary, and more research is needed to understand the direct effects of the carnivore diet on skin health. That said, certain nutrients play key roles in promoting skin health. These include:

- **Vitamin A:** This vitamin supports skin cell growth, repair, and maintenance. It helps regulate oil production, promotes the formation of healthy skin cells, and can aid in reducing acne. Vitamin A can be obtained from both animal sources (retinol) and plant sources (beta-carotene).

- **Vitamin C:** As a powerful antioxidant, vitamin C protects the skin from oxidative damage caused by free radicals. It is essential for collagen synthesis, which helps maintain skin elasticity and reduces the appearance of wrinkles. Vitamin C also aids in wound healing and brightens the skin.

- **Vitamin E:** Another potent antioxidant, vitamin E protects the skin from damage caused by environmental factors, such as UV radiation. It helps moisturize and strengthen the skin barrier, improving overall skin texture and reducing the appearance of scars and wrinkles.

- **Vitamin D:** While primarily known for its role in bone health, vitamin D also plays a role in skin health. It helps regulate cell growth and repair, enhances skin barrier function, and may have anti-inflammatory effects. Vitamin D can be synthesized by the body when the skin is exposed to sunlight or obtained from dietary sources.

- **B Vitamins:** B vitamins, such as niacin (B3), riboflavin (B2), and pantothenic acid (B5), contribute to healthy skin by promoting cell metabolism and supporting the production of energy and new skin cells. They also help maintain skin hydration and improve the skin's natural barrier function.

- **Vitamin K:** Vitamin K plays a crucial role in blood clotting, which can aid in wound healing and reduce the appearance of bruises and dark circles under the eyes. It may also have anti-inflammatory properties.

33. Is the Carnivore Diet Beneficial for Joint Health?

Joint health is influenced by a variety of factors, including genetics, age, lifestyle, physical activity, and nutrition. A well-rounded diet that provides essential nutrients is crucial for maintaining healthy joints.

The specific impact of the carnivore diet on joint health is not extensively studied, and there is a lack of official scientific evidence to support its effectiveness in improving or worsening joint conditions. Individual experiences may vary, and more research is needed to understand the direct effects of the carnivore diet on joint health.

Certain nutrients play a vital role in supporting joint health. For example, protein is essential for the maintenance and repair of connective tissues, including cartilage. Animal-based foods are the best, most bioavailable sources of dietary protein. Omega-3 fatty acids, primarily found in fatty fish, have potent anti-inflammatory benefits and may help reduce joint inflammation and pain. Minerals like calcium, magnesium, and phosphorus are important for bone health, which indirectly affects joint health.

However, while the carnivore diet provides important nutrients for joint health, it is important to consider potential concerns. The complete exclusion of plant-based foods may limit the intake of certain anti-inflammatory compounds found in fruits, vegetables, nuts, and seeds, which have been associated with joint health benefits. These may include compounds such as antioxidants and polyphenols. Antioxidants help reduce oxidative stress and inflammation in the body, which can benefit joint health. Fruits and vegetables, particularly brightly colored ones, are rich in various antioxidants, such as vitamin C, vitamin E, and beta-carotene (provitamin A). Additionally, certain plant-based foods contain polyphenols, which are bioactive compounds known for their anti-inflammatory properties. Polyphenols found in foods like berries, green tea, and spices have been linked to reduced inflammation and improved joint function.

Furthermore, an excessive intake of certain animal proteins and fats may contribute to inflammation in some individuals, potentially affecting joint health. Each person's joint health is unique, and dietary interventions can have different effects on individuals. Some individuals may experience improvements in joint conditions, such as reduced pain or inflammation, while others may not see significant changes or may even experience negative effects.

Typically, maintaining healthy joints involves a comprehensive approach that includes not only nutrition but also regular physical activity, weight management, proper joint biomechanics, and overall healthy lifestyle practices. While diet plays an important role in joint health, it should be considered as part of a holistic approach to joint care.

34. Is the Carnivore Diet Beneficial for Hormonal Health?

Hormonal health is a complex and intricate system that involves the interaction of numerous hormones and their delicate balance within the body. While the carnivore diet's impact on hormonal health has not been extensively studied, it is important to consider the potential mechanisms through which this dietary approach may influence hormones.

The carnivore diet places a significant emphasis on animal-based proteins and fats, which are rich sources of essential nutrients involved in hormone production and regulation. Proteins provide the building blocks for hormones, including amino acids necessary for the synthesis of various hormones, such as insulin, growth hormone, and thyroid hormones. Fats, particularly saturated and monounsaturated fats found in animal-based foods, are important for the production of steroid hormones, including testosterone, estrogen, and cortisol.

Additionally, the carnivore diet eliminates processed foods, refined carbohydrates, and potential allergens, which may help reduce inflammation and improve metabolic function. Chronic inflammation and metabolic dysregulation can disrupt hormonal balance and contribute to various hormonal disorders.

Hormonal health is influenced by a multiplicity of factors beyond just diet, such as lifestyle, stress levels, sleep quality, and individual physiology. Factors such as age, gender, underlying medical conditions, gut health, and genetic predispositions can also significantly impact hormonal balance.

Monitoring hormonal health while following the carnivore diet is oftentimes necessary, as prolonged adherence to a strict dietary approach may have unintended consequences on hormone production and balance. Regular assessment of hormone levels, such as testosterone, estrogen, thyroid hormones, and cortisol, can help ensure that any potential imbalances or deficiencies are detected and addressed promptly.

Overall, while the carnivore diet's influence on hormonal health is not extensively studied, it may have some benefits, as it provides essential nutrients involved in hormone production and regulation (in an extremely bioavailable form). However, individual needs, genetic factors, and overall lifestyle should also be considered, and consultations with healthcare professionals or registered dieticians are recommended to ensure personalized and well-informed dietary choices that support optimal hormonal health.

35. Is the Carnivore Diet Beneficial for Hypothyroidism?

Hypothyroidism is a condition characterized by an underactive thyroid gland, which leads to reduced production of thyroid hormones T4 (thyroxine) and T3 (triiodothyronine), which are responsible for regulating metabolism and various bodily functions. The role of the carnivore diet in managing hypothyroidism is not well-established and requires careful consideration of individual needs and underlying causes of the condition.

The carnivore diet's emphasis on animal-based proteins and fats can provide essential nutrients that are important for thyroid function. Animal proteins contain amino acids necessary for the synthesis of thyroid hormones, while fats, especially those found in animal sources, play an important role in hormone production and regulation. Additionally, the elimination of processed foods and potential allergens may help reduce inflammation, which can be beneficial for individuals with autoimmune-related hypothyroidism (e.g. Hashimoto's disease).

However, it is crucial to recognize that hypothyroidism is a complex condition influenced by multiple factors. Nutrient deficiencies, particularly iodine, selenium, zinc, iron, L-tyrosine, and vitamin C, can negatively affect thyroid function. It is important to ensure that the carnivore diet (or any diet you follow) provides adequate amounts of these nutrients through bioavailable food sources or, if necessary, supplementation. Here are some important key points about these nutrients:

- **Iodine:** Iodine is an essential mineral that plays a critical role in maintaining thyroid health by supporting the production of thyroid hormones, specifically thyroxine (T4) and triiodothyronine (T3).

Adequate iodine intake is vital for the proper functioning of the thyroid gland. Including dietary sources rich in iodine is crucial for individuals with hypothyroidism. Some excellent sources of iodine include iodized salt, which is a common staple in many households. Seaweed, such as kelp and nori, is another valuable source of iodine, providing a natural and nutrient-dense option.

Seafood, particularly fish and shellfish, is renowned for its iodine content and offers a delicious way to incorporate this essential mineral into the diet. Additionally, dairy products like milk, yogurt, and cheese can contribute to iodine intake, making them beneficial for individuals with hypothyroidism.

- **Selenium:** Selenium is a vital trace mineral that plays a crucial role in supporting thyroid function and overall thyroid health. It is an essential component of the enzymes involved in the metabolism of thyroid hormones, ensuring their proper synthesis, activation, and conversion within the body. Additionally, selenium acts as a potent antioxidant, helping to protect the thyroid gland from oxidative damage and inflammation.

Incorporating dietary sources rich in selenium is essential for individuals with hypothyroidism. Brazil nuts are particularly renowned for their high selenium content, providing an excellent natural source of this trace mineral. Seafood, including fish and shellfish, is another valuable dietary source of selenium. Meats like beef, pork, and poultry, as well as eggs, are additional sources of selenium that can be included in a well-balanced diet.

- **Zinc:** Zinc is an essential mineral that plays a vital role in the regulation of thyroid hormone synthesis and conversion. It is involved in various enzymatic reactions that support the proper functioning of the thyroid gland. Adequate zinc levels are essential for the production, activation, and utilization of thyroid hormones.

Including food sources rich in bioavailable zinc is important for individuals with hypothyroidism. Oysters, known for their high zinc content, are an excellent natural source of this essential mineral. Additionally, meats like beef, bison, and lamb are notable dietary sources of zinc, providing not only a savory taste but also a nutrient-dense option to support thyroid health.

By incorporating these zinc-rich foods into the diet, individuals with hypothyroidism can ensure optimal zinc levels, promoting proper thyroid hormone metabolism and overall thyroid function

- **Iron:** Iron is an essential mineral that plays a critical role in the production and regulation of thyroid hormones. It is a key component of proteins involved in thyroid hormone synthesis and metabolism, ensuring their proper function within the body.

Including dietary sources rich in iron is important for individuals with hypothyroidism. Red meat, such as beef and lamb, is an excellent source of heme iron, which is highly bioavailable and easily absorbed by the body. Poultry, including chicken and turkey, is another good source of iron. Seafood, particularly shellfish like oysters and clams, provides a nutrient-dense option for obtaining iron. Additionally, organ meats, especially liver, are known for their high iron content and can be incorporated into the diet to boost iron levels.

Maintaining adequate iron levels is crucial for optimal thyroid function and overall well-being. Iron supports the production of thyroid hormones and contributes to their regulation, ensuring a properly functioning thyroid gland. However, it is important to note that excessive iron intake can be harmful, so it is advisable to consult with a healthcare professional to determine individual iron needs and ensure appropriate intake.

By including iron-rich foods in the diet, individuals with hypothyroidism can support the intricate processes involved in thyroid hormone production and regulation, promoting optimal thyroid function and overall health.

• **L-tyrosine:** L-tyrosine is a vital amino acid that serves as a building block for the production of thyroid hormones. It plays a crucial role in the synthesis of thyroxine (T4) and triiodothyronine (T3), the key hormones produced by the thyroid gland.

Obtaining L-tyrosine from dietary sources is important for individuals with hypothyroidism. Protein-rich foods such as meat, including beef, pork, and lamb, provide a natural source of L-tyrosine. Poultry, such as chicken and turkey, is another excellent option. Fish, such as salmon and tuna, along with dairy products like milk, cheese, and yogurt, contribute to L-tyrosine intake. Eggs, a versatile and nutrient-dense food, also contain L-tyrosine.

By incorporating these protein-rich foods into the diet, individuals with hypothyroidism can support the production of thyroid hormones and promote optimal thyroid function.

- **Vitamin C:** Vitamin C is a powerful antioxidant and water-soluble vitamin that plays a crucial role in supporting the immune system and promoting overall health. It also aids in the absorption of iron, which is essential for proper thyroid function.

Including dietary sources rich in vitamin C is beneficial for individuals with hypothyroidism. Citrus fruits like oranges, grapefruits, and lemons are renowned for their high vitamin C content. Berries such as strawberries, blueberries, and raspberries are also excellent sources. Kiwi, peppers (particularly red and yellow varieties), and leafy green vegetables like spinach and kale are additional nutrient-dense options that provide vitamin C.

By incorporating these vitamin C-rich foods into the diet, individuals with hypothyroidism can support their immune system and optimize the absorption of iron, which is vital for thyroid health. It is important to note that vitamin C is easily destroyed by heat and oxygen, so consuming these foods in their fresh, raw, or lightly cooked form can help maximize vitamin C intake.

In cases where hypothyroidism has autoimmune origins, dietary interventions alone may not be sufficient to address the underlying autoimmunity. Managing autoimmune hypothyroidism involves a comprehensive approach that includes medical interventions, such as thyroid hormone replacement therapy (i.e. Synthroid®), and lifestyle modifications to support overall health and immune system function.

Individuals with hypothyroidism should work closely with healthcare professionals, such as endocrinologists or registered dietitians, who specialize in thyroid disorders. These professionals can assess individual needs, monitor thyroid function through appropriate testing, and provide personalized recommendations for dietary management. Regular monitoring of thyroid hormone levels and clinical symptoms is essential to ensure optimal management of hypothyroidism.

36. Is the Carnivore Diet Good for IBS?

Irritable bowel syndrome (IBS) is a common gastrointestinal disorder characterized by abdominal pain, bloating, and changes in bowel habits. While the effects of the carnivore diet on IBS are not fully established, there are certain aspects of the diet that may provide benefits for individuals with this condition. Understanding these factors can help evaluate the potential impact of the carnivore diet on IBS symptoms. Here are some important key points to consider:

- **Elimination of Potential Triggers:** The carnivore diet excludes several foods commonly associated with gastrointestinal symptoms in individuals with IBS, such as grains, legumes, and specific vegetables containing FODMAPs (fermentable oligosaccharides, disaccharides, monosaccharides, and polyols). FODMAPs are fermentable carbohydrates that can lead to excessive gas production and discomfort in some individuals. By removing these potential triggers, the carnivore diet may help reduce gastrointestinal irritation and inflammation, leading to improved symptoms for a lot of individuals.

• **Easier Digestion:** The carnivore diet emphasizes animal-based protein sources, which are generally easier for the digestive system to break down and absorb compared to plant-based proteins. This can be particularly beneficial for individuals with IBS as it may reduce the strain on the digestive system, potentially alleviating symptoms like bloating and discomfort.

• **Bioavailability of Nutrients:** Animal proteins are known for their high bioavailability, meaning that the body can efficiently absorb and utilize the nutrients they provide. This is especially important for individuals with IBS, as malabsorption of nutrients is oftentimes a concern. By consuming animal-based proteins, individuals with IBS may have a better chance of obtaining essential amino acids and other vital nutrients necessary for optimal health and well-being.

Overall, while the effects of the carnivore diet on IBS are still being studied, certain aspects of the diet, such as the elimination of potential triggers and the emphasis on easily digestible and bioavailable animal proteins, can offer benefits for some individuals. If you are an IBS sufferer and other diets have not worked for your condition, the carnivore diet is definitely one of the diets worth considering.

37. Is the Carnivore Diet Good for Psoriasis, Eczema, and Other Autoimmune Skin Conditions?

Psoriasis, eczema, and other autoimmune skin conditions are chronic inflammatory disorders characterized by skin inflammation, redness, itching, and discomfort. The impact of the carnivore diet on these conditions is not well-established and requires further scientific investigation. However, anecdotal reports suggest that some individuals with psoriasis, eczema, or other autoimmune skin conditions have experienced improvements in their symptoms while following the carnivore diet.

The carnivore diet's elimination of potential food triggers, such as grains, legumes, nuts, seeds, and certain vegetables, may reduce inflammation and alleviate symptoms in certain cases. These food groups are known to contain substances that can contribute to systemic inflammation and immunostimulation in susceptible individuals, such as anti-nutrients (i.e. lectins) and plant-defence compounds (i.e. alkaloids). By removing these potential dietary triggers, the carnivore diet may help reduce overall inflammation, which could potentially benefit individuals with autoimmune skin conditions.

Moreover, the carnivore diet's emphasis on high-quality, bioavailable, animal-based protein sources provides essential nutrients necessary for skin health, such as amino acids, vitamins (including vitamin D), minerals, and trace elements. These nutrients play important roles in skin structure, immune function, and wound healing. Adequate protein intake is particularly important for skin health, as proteins are essential for the production of collagen and other structural components of the skin.

38. Is the Carnivore Diet Anti-inflammatory?

The impact of the carnivore diet on inflammation is a hot topic of discussion. While some individuals have reported reduced inflammation and improved symptoms while following the carnivore diet, its overall anti-inflammatory effects are not well-established. Inflammation is a natural immune response that plays a critical role in the body's defence against infection and/or injury. However, chronic inflammation is associated with the development and progression of various diseases, including cardiovascular disease, diabetes, cancer, and autoimmune disorders.

Animal-based foods, which are the foundation of the carnivore diet, contain nutrients that can both promote and dampen inflammation, depending on various factors.

For example, certain nutrients found in animal products, such as omega-3 fatty acids and antioxidants, have been shown to have anti-inflammatory properties. Omega-3 fatty acids, primarily obtained from fatty fish and seafood, have been associated with reduced inflammation and improved inflammatory biomarkers in the blood. Similarly, antioxidants found in animal-based foods, such as vitamin E and selenium, can counteract oxidative stress and inflammation.

On the other opposite side, animal-based foods also contain compounds that can promote inflammation. For example, red meat and processed meats have been associated with increased levels of inflammatory markers in some studies. These meats contain compounds like heme iron, certain types of saturated fats, and when overcooked, compounds like heterocyclic amines (HCAs), polycyclic aromatic hydrocarbons (PAHs), and advanced glycation end products (AGEs), which have been linked with the onset of inflammation and oxidative stress.

The impact of the carnivore diet on inflammation may vary among individuals. Factors such as genetic predisposition, existing health conditions, and overall dietary balance can influence the body's inflammatory response to the diet. Additionally, the duration and adherence to the carnivore diet may also play a role in its impact on inflammation.

To gain a better understanding of how the carnivore diet affects inflammation, further research is needed. Well-controlled studies that assess inflammation markers and clinical outcomes in individuals following the diet are necessary for accurate conclusions.

39. Why is the Carnivore Diet Considered an Elimination Diet?

The carnivore diet is oftentimes considered an elimination diet because it involves the elimination of a wide range of foods that are commonly associated with inflammation, allergies, intolerances, and sensitivities. By excluding potentially problematic foods such as grains, legumes, nuts, seeds, and certain vegetables, the carnivore diet aims to eliminate potential triggers and allow individuals to observe the impact of specific foods on their symptoms and overall well-being.

Elimination diets are commonly used in clinical practice to identify food intolerances and sensitivities, which can manifest as a variety of symptoms such as digestive issues, skin problems, headaches, mental health issues, sleep problems, and fatigue. These symptoms can be caused by various physiological mechanisms, including immune-mediated responses, enzyme deficiencies, or disturbances in gut function.

By eliminating a broad range of foods and then gradually reintroducing them one at a time, individuals following the carnivore diet can observe any changes in their symptoms and identify specific foods that may be contributing to their health issues. This process allows for the identification of potential food triggers and the customization of the diet based on individual tolerances and sensitivities.

40. Is the Carnivore Diet Good for Autism?

The impact of the carnivore diet on autism is a topic that has not been extensively researched, and the available scientific evidence is quite limited. Autism spectrum disorder (ASD) is a complex neurodevelopmental condition characterized by challenges in social interaction, communication, and repetitive behaviors. It is influenced by a combination of genetic, environmental, and neurological factors.

Dietary interventions for autism have gained attention as potential adjunctive therapies, aiming to alleviate symptoms and improve overall well-being. However, it is important to approach these interventions with caution and in collaboration with healthcare professionals who specialize in autism spectrum disorders.

While anecdotal reports and individual accounts may suggest improvements in certain symptoms with the carnivore diet, it is crucial to recognize that autism is a multifaceted condition, and dietary interventions alone may not address the core deficits associated with ASD. The effects of diet on autism symptoms can vary widely among individuals, and what works for one person may not work for another.

When considering dietary interventions for autism, it is essential to adopt a comprehensive and individualized approach. This includes taking into account the specific nutritional needs of the individual, considering any sensory sensitivities or aversions to certain foods, and ensuring that the diet provides a balanced and varied nutrient profile.

41. Is the Carnivore Diet Beneficial for People With Multiple Food Allergies and Sensitivities?

Yes. The carnivore diet can be beneficial for individuals with multiple food allergies and sensitivities due to its exclusion of irritating plant compounds and its emphasis on bioavailable animal protein, specifically collagen and gelatin found in animal-based foods. These components support gut health and contribute to the healing and sealing of the gut lining.

The gut lining plays a crucial role in preventing the passage of undigested food particles and potentially harmful substances into the bloodstream, which can trigger immune responses and food sensitivities. By consuming animal protein, individuals following the carnivore diet can provide their bodies with the necessary amino acids, such as proline and glycine, which are important building blocks for collagen production.

Collagen is the most abundant structural protein in the human body. It is a key component of connective tissues, which provide strength, support, and structure to various parts of the body. Collagen makes up a significant portion of the skin, bones, tendons, ligaments, and cartilage. It also helps maintain the integrity of the gut lining and supports gut barrier function. By supporting the health of the gut lining, collagen can help reduce the risk of food particles crossing into the bloodstream and triggering allergic or sensitivity reactions.

It is worth noting that while the carnivore diet may provide benefits for individuals with multiple food allergies, sensitivities, and intolerances, it is still essential to work with healthcare professionals, such as allergists or registered dietitians, to ensure proper nutrient intake and to develop a well-balanced and individualized diet plan. Additionally, it is crucial to address any underlying health conditions and to consider other factors that may contribute to allergies and sensitivities, such as environmental triggers and immune dysregulation.

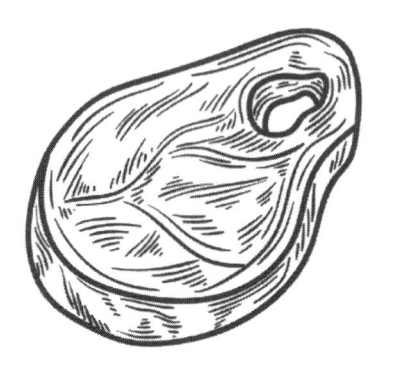

CONCLUSION

Final Thoughts and Future Directions

The carnivore diet is a simple, minimalistic, yet powerful dietary approach for improving health and wellness outcomes. It's a diet based entirely on animal products, especially meat (i.e. beef, lamb, bison, poultry, pork, etc). Eggs and dairy products are also included depending on the carnivore diet variation and strictness. Fatty cuts of meat, such as ribeye, New York strip, Delmonico, etc, and organ meats (offal), such as liver, heart, and spleen, are particularly desirable in the diet due to their micronutrient density.

The primary goal of the carnivore diet is to restore health and vitality to the body by addressing nutrient deficiencies and eliminating inflammatory foods that may irritate the gut and stimulate the immune system. Some people call the carnivore diet a "zero-carb diet" because it eliminates all sources of carbohydrates. This is especially true when the diet is comprised only of meat (e.g. meat-only diet).

Many people consider carnivore to be a more extreme version of the ketogenic diet, which also includes very few carbohydrates and emphasizes nutrient-dense, whole foods. Anecdotally, the carnivore diet has shown great potential in healing gut permeability, also known as "leaky gut syndrome," which is a primary etiological factor in autoimmunity.

The mainstream medical world is quite resistant to accepting leaky gut syndrome as a leading contributor to autoimmune diseases. Despite that, autoimmune patients from all over the world try the carnivore diet and see the results for themselves. There are so many amazing stories out there that it's simply hard to deny the evidence. The diet works, and it works very well.

By eating 100% strict carnivore, individuals are able to finally eliminate the majority of dietary toxins and antigens—both synthetic and natural—that could otherwise irritate their gut and stimulate their immune system. The carnivore diet supplies the body with an abundance of essential macro- and micronutrients, such as amino acids, fatty acids, cholesterol, minerals, trace elements, enzymes, and other co-factors not found in plant-based foods. These dietary constituents are crucial for restoring proper gut function, immune health, and overall well-being.

Future scientific studies, reports, and interventions will hopefully shed light on why and how the carnivore diet is so effective at managing, reversing, and even healing "incurable" chronic conditions.

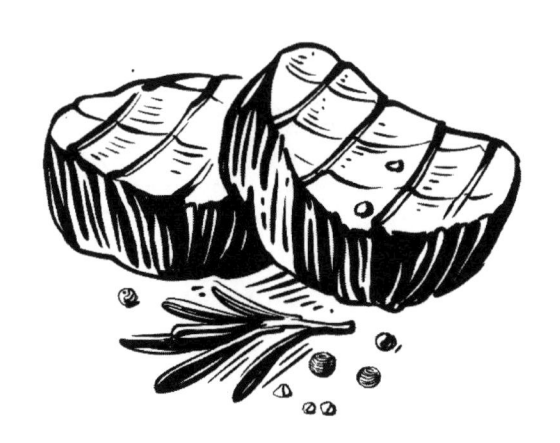

Your Opinion Matters

Did this book help you in some way?
If so, we'd love to hear about it!
Scan the QR code below to leave your honest review.

Scan here!

About The Author

Dr. Christopher Shaw is a distinguished nutritionist and naturopathic doctor with a big passion for guiding individuals towards a healthier way of life through informed nutritional decisions and lifestyle habits. Possessing an extensive wealth of knowledge and an unyielding commitment to personalized well-being, Dr. Shaw has emerged as a respected figure in the domain of natural health and alternative medicine.

His evidence-based methodology, coupled with a compassionate and empathetic approach, has made him a sought-after authority in the fields of nutrition and natural health. Through his expertise, he empowers clients and patients to develop long-lasting habits that foster optimized health, vitality, and wellness.

References

Chapter 1

1. Megan R. Ruth et al., *"Consuming a hypocaloric high-fat low carbohydrate diet for 12 weeks lowers C-reactive protein, and raises serum adiponectin and high-density lipoprotein-cholesterol in obese subjects,"* Metabolism. 2013 Dec; 62(12): 10.1016/j.metabol.2013.07.006.

2. Tara Kelly et al., *"Low-Carbohydrate Diets in the Management of Obesity and Type 2 Diabetes: A Review from Clinicians Using the Approach in Practice,"* Int J Environ Res Public Health. 2020 Apr; 17(7): 2557. Published online 2020 Apr 8.

3. Lisa Quigley et al., *"The complex microbiota of raw milk,"* FEMS Microbiology Reviews, Volume 37, Issue 5, September 2013, Pages 664–698.

4. Dominik H Pesta et al., *"A high-protein diet for reducing body fat: mechanisms and possible caveats,"* Nutr Metab (Lond). 2014; 11: 53. Published online 2014 Nov 19.

5. Jaecheol Moon et al., *"Clinical Evidence and Mechanisms of High-Protein Diet-Induced Weight Loss,"* J Obes Metab Syndr. 2020 Sep 30; 29(3): 166–173. Published online 2020 Jul 23.

6. Mona Mohamed Ibrahim Abdalla, *"Ghrelin – Physiological Functions and Regulation,"* Eur Endocrinol. 2015 Aug; 11(2): 90–95. Published online 2015 Aug 19.

7. David Furman et al., *"Chronic inflammation in the etiology of disease across the life span,"* Nat Med. 2019 Dec; 25(12): 1822–1832. Published online 2019 Dec 5.

8. Roma Pahwa et al., *"Chronic Inflammation,"* StatPearls [Internet].

9. Robert Oh et al., *"Low Carbohydrate Diet,"* StatPearls [Internet].

10. Insaf Berrazaga et al., *"The Role of the Anabolic Properties of Plant- versus Animal-Based Protein Sources in Supporting Muscle Mass Maintenance: A Critical Review,"* Nutrients. 2019 Aug; 11(8): 1825. Published online 2019 Aug 7.

11. Andrew J. Murray et al., *"Novel ketone diet enhances physical and cognitive performance,"* FASEB J. 2016 Dec; 30(12): 4021–4032. Published online 2016 Aug 15.

12. Kristin L. Osterberg et al., *"Carbohydrate exerts a mild influence on fluid retention following exercise-induced dehydration,"* J Appl Physiol (1985) . 2010 Feb;108(2):245-50.

Chapter 2

1. L. Wyness et al., *"Red meat in the diet: an update,"* Nutrition Bulletin, 16 February 2011 https://doi.org/10.1111/j.1467-3010.2010.01871.

2. Matthew G. Dunnigan et al., *"An epidemiological model of privational rickets and osteomalacia,"* Cambridge University Press: 28 February 2007.

3. Sarah K. Gebauer et al., *"Effects of Ruminant trans Fatty Acids on Cardiovascular Disease and Cancer: A Comprehensive Review of Epidemiological, Clinical, and Mechanistic Studies,"* Advances in Nutrition, Volume 2, Issue 4, July 2011, Pages 332–354.\

4. Sinéad Weldon et al., *"Conjugated linoleic acid and atherosclerosis: no effect on molecular markers of cholesterol homeostasis in THP-1 macrophages,"* Atherosclerosis Volume 174, Issue 2, June 2004, Pages 261-273.

5. J.W. Ryder et al., *"Isomer-Specific Antidiabetic Properties of Conjugated Linoleic Acid,"* Diabetes 2001 May; 50(5): 1149-1157.

6. Nelsy Castro-Webb et al., *"Cross-sectional study of conjugated linoleic acid in adipose tissue and risk of diabetes,"* Am J Clin Nutr. 2012 Jul;96(1):175-81.

7. Martha A Belury et al., *"Conjugated linoleic acid is an activator and ligand for peroxisome proliferator-activated receptor-gamma (PPARγ),"* Nutrition Research Volume 22, Issue 7, July 2002, Pages 817-824.

8. Julio J Ochoa et al., *"Conjugated linoleic acids (CLAs) decrease prostate cancer cell proliferation: different molecular mechanisms for cis-9, trans-11 and trans-10, cis-12 isomers,"* Carcinogenesis. 2004 Jul;25(7):1185-91.

9. Zeneng Wang et al., *"Gut flora metabolism of phosphatidylcholine promotes cardiovascular disease,"* Nature. 2011 Apr 7;472(7341):57-63.

10. Loren Cordain et al., *"Origins and evolution of the Western diet: health implications for the 21st century,"* Am J Clin Nutr. 2005 Feb;81(2):341-54.

11. Renata Micha et al., *"Red and processed meat consumption and risk of incident coronary heart disease, stroke, and diabetes: A systematic review and meta-analysis,"* Circulation. 2010 Jun 1; 121(21): 2271–2283.

12. T J Key et al., *"Dietary habits and mortality in 11,000 vegetarians and health conscious people: results of a 17 year follow up,"* BMJ. 1996 Sep 28;313(7060):775-9.

13. Gwyneth K Davey et al., *"EPIC-Oxford: lifestyle characteristics and nutrient intakes in a cohort of 33 883 meat-eaters and 31 546 non meat-eaters in the UK,"* Public Health Nutr. 2003 May;6(3):259-69.

14. Peter J. Turnbaugh et al., *"The Effect of Diet on the Human Gut Microbiome: A Metagenomic Analysis in Humanized Gnotobiotic Mice,"* Sci Transl Med. 2009 Nov 11; 1(6): 6ra14.

Chapter 3

1. Wajeed Masood et al., *"Ketogenic Diet,"* StatPearls.

2. Susan A. Masino et al., *"Mechanisms of Ketogenic Diet Action,"* National Center for Biotechnology Information (US); 2012.

3. Giovanna Muscogiuri et al., *"The management of very low-calorie ketogenic diet in obesity outpatient clinic: a practical guide,"* J Transl Med. 2019; 17: 356. Published online 2019 Oct 29.

4. Victoria M. Gershuni et al., *"Nutritional Ketosis for Weight Management and Reversal of Metabolic Syndrome,"* Curr Nutr Rep. 2018 Sep; 7(3): 97–106.

5. Adriano Bruci et al., *"Very Low-Calorie Ketogenic Diet: A Safe and Effective Tool for Weight Loss in Patients with Obesity and Mild Kidney Failure,"* Nutrients. 2020 Feb; 12(2): 333. Published online 2020 Jan 27.

Chapter 4

1. David O. Kennedy, *"B Vitamins and the Brain: Mechanisms, Dose and Efficacy—A Review,"* Nutrients. 2016 Feb; 8(2): 68. Published online 2016 Jan 28.

2. Adarsh Kumar et al., *"Role of coenzyme Q10 (CoQ10) in cardiac disease, hypertension and Meniere-like syndrome,"* Pharmacol Ther . 2009 Dec;124(3):259-68.

3. Mario Festin et al., *"Nausea and vomiting in early pregnancy,"* BMJ Clin Evid. 2009; 2009: 1405. Published online 2009 Jun 3.

4. F L Santos et al, *"Systematic review and meta-analysis of clinical trials of the effects of low carbohydrate diets on cardiovascular risk factors,"* Obes Rev . 2012 Nov;13(11):1048-66.

5. Luc Djoussé et al., *"Dietary cholesterol and coronary artery disease: a systematic review,"* Curr Atheroscler Rep . 2009 Nov;11(6):418-22.

6. Ronald P Mensink et al., *"Effects of dietary fatty acids and carbohydrates on the ratio of serum total to HDL cholesterol and on serum lipids and apolipoproteins: a meta-analysis of 60 controlled trials,"* Am J Clin Nutr. 2003 May;77(5):1146-55.

7. Allon N. Friedman et al., *"Independent influence of dietary protein on markers of kidney function and disease in obesity,"* Kidney International Volume 78, Issue 7, 1 October 2010, Pages 693-697.

8. Helga Frank et al., *"Effect of short-term high-protein compared with normal-protein diets on renal hemodynamics and associated variables in healthy young men,"* Am J Clin Nutr. 2009 Dec;90(6):1509-16.

9. Stephen P. Juraschek et al., *"Effect of a High-Protein Diet on Kidney Function in Healthy Adults: Results From the OmniHeart Trial,"* Am J Kidney Dis. 2013 April; 61(4): 547–554.

10. William F Martin et al., *"Dietary protein intake and renal function,"* Nutr Metab (Lond). 2005; 2: 25.

11. Allon N Friedman et al., *"Comparative effects of low-carbohydrate high-protein versus low-fat diets on the kidney,"* Clin J Am Soc Nephrol. 2012 Jul;7(7):1103-11.

12. Hercules Sakkas et al., *"Nutritional Status and the Influence of the Vegan Diet on the Gut Microbiota and Human Health,"* Medicina (Kaunas). 2020 Feb; 56(2): 88. Published online 2020 Feb 22.

Printed in Great Britain
by Amazon